midwife pip's
Guide to a Positive Birth

midwife pip's

Guide to a
Positive Birth

TOOLS TO FEEL CALM
AND CONFIDENT

Pip Davies

Vermilion
LONDON

1

Vermilion, an imprint of Ebury Publishing
20 Vauxhall Bridge Road
London SW1V 2SA

Vermilion is part of the Penguin Random House group of companies
whose addresses can be found at global.penguinrandomhouse.com

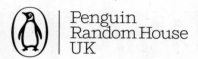

Copyright © Pip Davies 2024
Illustrations by Emily Voller

Pip Davies has asserted her right to be identified as the author of this Work
in accordance with the Copyright, Designs and Patents Act 1988

First published by Vermilion in 2024

www.penguin.co.uk

A CIP catalogue record for this book is available from the British Library

ISBN 9781785044786

Typeset in 11/15.5 pt Baskerville MT Pro by Jouve (UK), Milton Keynes
Printed and bound in Great Britain by Clays Ltd, Elcograf S.p.A.

The authorised representative in the EEA is Penguin Random House Ireland,
Morrison Chambers, 32 Nassau Street, Dublin D02 YH68

Penguin Random House is committed to a sustainable
future for our business, our readers and our planet. This
book is made from Forest Stewardship Council® certified paper.

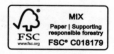

For all the women with babies in their hearts, wombs or arms.
You are stronger than you think and more capable than you realise.
I hope this book allows you to recognise how incredible you
are and empowers you on your journey.

CONTENTS

INTRODUCTION

Welcome to *Midwife Pip's Guide to a Positive Birth*. Through these pages I will hold your hand along this incredible journey and provide you with everything you need to welcome your baby into the world in a positive, empowering way, regardless of what that looks like for you and your little one.

Before I immerse you in all things birth and baby preparation, I'd like to introduce myself. I am Pip, 'Midwife Pip', experienced practising midwifery sister, MSc graduate, founder of the *Midwife Pip Podcast*, hypnobirth and antenatal educator, pre- and postnatal exercise trainer, Mummy MOT practitioner and, most importantly, a mum. Having worked in midwifery for over a decade in various roles and settings – from low-risk birthing centres and antenatal and postnatal wards, to assessment units, in the community, home births and, more recently, as a labour ward coordinator and midwifery sister – I have witnessed first-hand how so many families are poorly equipped with conflicting, inaccurate or unrealistic advice and information when it comes to birth.

I LOVE being a midwife. I truly believe I have the most wonderful job – every day I am able to witness birth, and each is unique and incredible in its own way. But, more than that, each day I support women in all their strength and courage as they become mothers; some for the first time, others for the tenth, but that moment is one that never tires in its beauty. The women I feel so blessed to support make me feel immensely proud to be a woman – watching everyday miracles and the strength that women hold never ceases to amaze me.

Just like those women I work with every day, you and I are in this book together, and I am so excited that you are joining me, because I know how important this time is for you. Pregnancy, birth and early motherhood are areas I am immensely (some say relentlessly) passionate about, and I have an ethos that all women deserve their birth to be the most empowering experience possible. Birth is more than just one day, it is the creation of memories that stay with us forever; it is the earliest influence on our start to motherhood and we need to ensure that, through comprehensive preparation, the journey of labour and birth is a positive one. Before we begin, I want you to recognise how worthy and important you are in this precious time of pregnancy. As you work through these chapters with me, I hope you will begin to truly understand how incredible and capable you are and how powerful we can be as women when we trust in our bodies and approach birth with a calm confidence and reliable information.

You are clearly invested in you and your baby because you have picked up this book and chosen to inform and empower yourself ahead of the most precious time in your life. In return, I am invested in providing you with a comprehensive understanding ahead of birth. You deserve the best and, after feeling the benefits of knowledge and empowerment during my own beautiful birth in 2021, I want you to also feel like a superwoman when you birth your baby. The reality is you cannot accurately predict or plan your birth – there are many variables and twists or turns that may crop up – but what you *can* do is prepare and get to know all of your options. My promise to you, after you finish reading this book, is that you will feel fully prepared for your own unique birth. It may feature some hiccups, but, by working through this guide with me, you will be equipped for these variables to help shape a positive experience even if things do not go according to plan A.

Through the journey of reading this book you will learn that you, and your body, are stronger and more capable than you realise.

WHY YOUR BIRTH PREPARATION MATTERS

You and your baby are the priority throughout this book – I have written every word, sentence and chapter to ensure you are psychologically and physically prepared for birth.

I want to explore the concept of a 'positive birth' because, when talking about a positive birth, I don't mean a certain *type* of birth, but, instead, a feeling. A positive birth may come in many forms; it may not be the birth you plan and yet you can still feel empowered by the experience and reflect on what you and your body achieved with positivity. The truth is, there is no one best way, no right or wrong way to birth your baby, and it is my mission to ensure you can navigate your journey with a calm confidence, to make informed choices and decisions for you and your baby.

Birth preparation matters. But the reality is that not all birth preparation is equal. The title of 'birth educator' or 'hypnobirthing teacher' can be obtained with very little expertise and training, and, as a midwife working in birth settings for years, I have seen many families who have been poorly prepared for birth through being misinformed or not educated on all the twists and turns of birth despite their best efforts to equip themselves with knowledge and understanding. This is not going to be the same for you – women deserve better, and I am gifting you reliable, evidenced-based information through this book. No matter what stage of pregnancy you are in, it is never too early or too late to begin your birth preparation.

Your birth experience – the way you feel the moment your little one is welcomed earthside – is much too important to leave to chance. If we compare birth preparation to the average wedding day preparation, there is often a huge disparity. You may have planned a wedding yourself, or watched others do so, but it is fair to say that wedding days often have at least a year of lead up, visiting venues, tasting food, planning, preparing, spending time and money to make it perfect; nothing is left to chance (of course I am generalising, but you get my point). The way you feel about growing and birthing your child will change you as a person forever and a positive birth will strengthen you in ways you can only imagine before it happens. Viewing your birth with a similar degree of thought and care is important to achieving your positive birth goals.

I would love everyone to really know what their body does and is capable of doing, to trust in its ability and to have education around how to best support your body and baby through the physiological process of labour. I have tried to cover as much of this essential information as possible, but, of course, every pregnancy is completely unique and you may find something arises in your own pregnancy that is outside of the scope of this book. In this case, I would always urge you to speak with your medical professional for any individualised medical advice.

Pregnancy is a powerful time to start prioritising your self-care when your body is dedicating so much of itself to growing your baby. It is about valuing yourself and building your own self-love and appreciation, and, by doing so, you can intuitively tap into the calm confidence within yourself that is needed for your birth.

Self-care is an important piece of your well-being in pregnancy, but please understand that self-care is not simply cooking yourself a nice meal or a taking a shower – these are basic human rights. Self-care is more than this, it is a level up – it is an undisturbed bubble bath, a walk in nature, five minutes to breathe calmly in your room. Small acts of self-care are achievable in everyday life, and we must seize them, schedule them and never feel guilty about them.

Practising self-care in pregnancy is a powerful gift you can give to your growing baby.

Before you begin on your pregnancy and parenting journey, I invite you to make some promises to yourself, to benefit yourself in pregnancy as well as your baby. Below are five promises to make to yourself on this journey. Feel free to come up with some of your own or stick with mine – it's up to you. You may wish to write these on a Post-it note to stick on the mirror where you brush your teeth or on the fridge door – somewhere you can see them – to keep reminding yourself.

I promise to . . .

1. Prioritise my well-being without apology or guilt.
2. Calmly and confidently ask questions.
3. Not compare myself to others.
4. Check in on my mindset daily.
5. Move and nourish my body and baby.

You cannot pour from an empty cup – if you are burned out, you are not going to be the present, patient parent you strive to be. We are human beings, not robots, and by filling up our cup we can fill up our children's cups too, but if we are empty, we have nothing to give. Loving, looking after and appreciating yourself will allow your child to learn to do the same – it is not a selfish act; it is essential for your family to thrive and to truly be well.

HOW TO USE THIS BOOK

If a positive and informed birth is your goal, then I am pleased to say that you are in exactly the right place. For you to get the very best from this book, I just want to highlight a few things.

First, this is so much more than a book; it is an interactive, supportive guide and I am here with you. There are pages for you to write on – writing on precious, freshly printed pages feels wrong, I know, but trust me, in optimising your birth it *is* right, so get yourself a pen! You will notice some 'Pause for Thought' sections at the end of some chapters and I encourage you to actively pause and consider these milestones and how you are feeling at each stage.

There is also a QR code for you here:

As you work through the book, you will see I refer to this code, as it links through to videos and other resources I have made especially for you to make sure we leave no stone unturned as you prepare for this journey. Give it a scan now and join our Community Support Group, where you will be able to connect with other expectant mums on the same journey as you. When women support women amazing things happen and, of course, I am in there too, so I look forward to saying 'Hello' soon.

I have broken this book into three parts:

- Part 1: Preparing For Your Birth
- Part 2: It's Time to Birth
- Part 3: You Did It: Immediately Post-Birth

I recommend reading the book in this order and engaging in the mini activities and practices throughout. In this way, the book becomes your guide, and I am able to support you step by step towards a positive birth outcome. You'll then be able to dip in and out of the book and revisit key topics and practices as you need to. While I have a chapter dedicated to birth partners, I would encourage them to read the whole book, too, so they also know what to expect and how to best support you.

Along the way, I have also included key points and messages from experts in the different areas to ensure you receive 360-degree insights about your care and options. We are going for a no-stone-unturned, fully comprehensive, judgement-free and compassionate approach to preparing you for this incredible journey. Are you ready to feel empowered?

PART 1
Preparing For Your Birth

Welcome to the start of your journey.

In this part, I will walk you through preparing your mind for birth, truly understanding your female anatomy and body (spoiler alert: you are INCREDIBLE), and how to prepare physically for your birth during your pregnancy. We will cover all the psychological and physical preparations you need to know about during pregnancy so that you are ready to boss your birth.

As we walk through Part 1, you will discover how powerfully you can influence your birth and be in control every step of the way. We will work together page by page to set the foundations for how you wish your birth to look and feel, and then explore how this can be flexed to fit different situations that could crop up. By the end of this part you will literally have your bags packed and be excited to dive into Part 2.

1

NURTURING YOUR MIND FOR AN EMPOWERED BIRTH

The connection between your mind and body is a powerful partnership that influences everything from pregnancy to how your body works during labour and beyond into the postpartum. I've therefore dedicated this first chapter to exploring how you can prepare your mind for birth.

How you currently feel about birthing your baby will be unique to you. Throughout this chapter, we will explore your current mindset and emotions and help you to realise just how capable you are of birthing your baby.

UNDERSTANDING THE MIND–BODY CONNECTION

Your incredible brain is neuroplastic, which means that it is able to adapt, continuously learn and rewire your thoughts, feelings and perceptions. Having this skill is very valuable during pregnancy as it means that you have the power to change the way you view birth, which is reassuring if you have birth fears that may form barriers to you having a calm and positive experience.

Your thoughts are not set in stone – you have the power to change them.

Your mind influences your physical body and the sensations you experience. Your mindset during labour is therefore important and is linked to your body's ability to produce the hormones that are crucial for bringing your little one into the world, such as oxytocin, the hormone responsible for labour starting and progressing. When your brain feels calm and safe, it can produce much more oxytocin than when it is in a place of anxiety or feels threatened – when it will suppress oxytocin and allow 'stress' hormones such as adrenaline and cortisol to dominate. These hormones inhibit contractions and therefore prevent labour from starting or continuing. This means, for your labour to begin and to progress smoothly, your mind needs to be in the right place too.

The optimal state for your brain to be in during labour mirrors the way your brain works when you are having sex. This is because when you are having (good) sex, your mind isn't thinking about what to add to the grocery list or the washing up left in the sink; your mind isn't really thinking at all in fact – you are simply relaxed and 'doing'. The practical, thinking part of your brain, called the neocortex, is dimmed, and the instinctive, mammalian part of your brain is turned up. This fine-tuning of your brain allows your mind to relax and your hormones to work optimally. When you achieve this during sex, it results in orgasm, and during labour it allows your body's natural physiology to take over and for birth to happen. This is why developing self-confidence and the ability to remove your conscious thinking brain and relax into the process of labour is a powerful tool. You need to be free enough to let go, to not overthink or overanalyse, to not worry, as this amplifies your practical brain again, signalling that there is a potential threat and labour needs to stop.

A mammal in the wild, for example, could be labouring away and then spot a predator – their adrenaline levels rise as they no longer feel safe to birth their offspring and they stop labouring. They have three options: fight, flight or freeze. In any of these options, their blood supply is directed to their limbs to allow them to get out of danger and directed away from their uterus or womb, which stops their contractions from happening. The same can happen to humans when labouring. In threatening situations, your mind is fearful and signals to your body that there is a perceived threat, and it is not safe to give birth. As a result, your energy and blood supply are directed to your arm and leg muscles to allow you to run away and escape from or fight off this threat, and the supply to your uterus is reduced so contractions slow or stop and labour stalls. This is a key survival instinct for animals in the wild to keep their offspring safe, but is less useful to us as birthing women in safe environments.

A relaxed mind translates into a relaxed body, and a relaxed, calm body is one which is prone to a more straightforward and comfortable birth.

Your body believes what your mind tells it – the two are so power-fully interconnected, which is why understanding this link and building your positive mindset is so valuable as you prepare for birth. Let me give you an example: you're in a mid-afternoon energy slump and are starting to feel hungry and think about your favourite treat – for me it's a big slice of carrot cake topped with butter cream icing (don't judge!). Without actually seeing or tasting it, your mind decides it is only that thing you have been imagining that will satisfy you – your mouth may even start to water. This is just one example of how your mind can physically influence your body and how it responds to sensations. To put this in the context of birth, if you understand your body and baby, and are not fearful of the sensations you experience, your body is physically able to relax and respond positively as a direct result of what you believe and imagine. Powerful stuff.

If you still need some convincing about just how intertwined our minds and bodies are, here is a small experiment to do. Ideally, close your eyes and ask someone to read this out to you. You can also complete this exercise live with me by scanning the QR code on page 6.

- Hold out both arms in front of you, straight, at shoulder height with palms facing downwards.
- In one hand, imagine you are clutching a bucket full of heavy, wet sand.
- In the other hand, imagine you are holding on to a bunch of light, airy balloons.
- Imagine gripping tighter to the bucket of very heavy, wet sand as I now add extra sand to the bucket, making it even heavier to hold.
- In your other hand, the balloons feel light, airy and comfortable to hold.
- More and more wet sand is added into the bucket. The bucket is heavier and harder to hold up now and you may even feel your arm being dragged down as you try to keep hold of it.
- The balloons are still light and airy, drifting upwards comfortably.
- Even more heavy wet sand is added to your bucket – you are really having to focus now to keep that bucket held up.
- Now open your eyes and look at your arms. It is highly likely you'll notice the arm you imagined holding the bucket of sand is lower than the one holding the balloons.

This is an important message as it demonstrates how what we tell our minds really does change the way our bodies behave physically too.

AFFIRMATIONS FOR BIRTH

I want to introduce you to the world of affirmations. You may be familiar with these already, but, either way, they are an easy, helpful tool for the journey of birth and parenthood you are about to embark on.

Affirmations are simply statements that support you to overcome negative thoughts and, when regularly read and repeated so you can believe them, they can empower you to create positive changes in your mind. A simple sequence of words can completely switch your mindset, turn a bad day into a good one, transform an anxious mind into a place of gratitude and calm and change a doubting mind into a confident, self-compassionate one. When you find that one that connects with you – wow, it is powerful.

Affirmations can be used whenever there's a want or need for you to create a positive change in your life. This could be anything causing feelings of self-doubt or anxiety and where you need to boost your self-confidence and self-esteem or overcome anxieties and frustrations. They work really well through many life events, such as a work presentation, a new exercise challenge and, of course . . . birth. I can also confirm they are a great tool for the whirlwind of motherhood too.

If you are wondering *'Do they really work?'* I have exciting news and the answer is a firm yes. Studies have actually proved that the use of affirmations can lead to people performing better at work, managing stress more effectively and even improving mental health conditions.

I will be popping some of my favourite affirmations for this time in your life throughout this book and encourage you to sit with them as they arise and see how they feel to you. Some will connect with you on a deeper level than others and this is perfectly normal as we are all individuals. A great idea is to also create your own affirmation: when a negative thought crops up, sit with it and think *'How would I support a friend with this negative belief?'* Write down your response and you may be surprised to realise you had the solution within you all along. I have shared a couple of examples of me trying out this same exercise:

Examples:

'I am appreciating my body just the way it is and am grateful to be healthy today.'

'It is OK to find this challenging, because it is challenging, but I am capable of overcoming challenges.'

Now you try it . . .

_____

_____

_____

_____

_____

_____

_____

_____

_____

PRACTICAL TOOLS TO PREPARE YOUR MIND

So much of labour and parenthood is influenced by our mindset, and we need to protect, prioritise and practise creating a 'can-do' positive mindset with the ability to be flexible and confident in the tools and techniques you will have when needed during birth. Let's start with exploring your current perceptions around birth.

Exploring your birth thoughts

Before I begin to help you plan your own positive birth, it's important to unpick and debunk common misconceptions about birth that may be getting in your way. This is very much a process, and we cannot wipe away all previous influences overnight, but we can seize regular opportunities to challenge our ideas around birth.

Far too many of us think of words such as 'fear' or 'anxiety' when we think about birth. But why is this? We are living in a time when birth is safer than ever before, so why are women more fearful of it? Approximately 80 per cent of women live with mild fear around birth and 10–20 per cent have a severe level of fear around birth.

If this is how you feel, remember you are not alone in these thoughts. With birth often dramatised in TV, films and the media, it is understandable that you may feel anxious, overwhelmed, nervous or even scared when you think about birth. But birth does not have to be this way – you can feel **calm**, **capable** and **excited** for your birth.

As a practising midwife I am blessed to have witnessed many truly positive births every day; each is a unique journey, but all are equally raw and beautiful. With the correct education, preparation and support, *all* women can have a positive and empowered birth experience. Whether you have a planned or unplanned caesarean birth, a water birth, an epidural birth, an assisted birth or use hypnobirthing, every single type of birth can be positive.

For as long as I can remember, I was always anxious and fearful about childbirth, not helped by the awful depictions of labour and birth on TV and in movies. Strangely, becoming pregnant brought a sense of calm over me, and the anxiety fell away. I felt birth was an almost inevitable out-come, so I should just get on with preparing as best as I could.

As a result of all my prep, I largely knew what to expect and felt calm and confident throughout pregnancy and birth. I was happy with the choices I made through pregnancy and understood the changes I felt as the baby grew bigger. And as it got to the final days, I knew to stay relaxed, distract myself and, when contractions started, to go to my happy place. And I knew exactly when to start pushing during labour. I trusted my body to do the right thing, and it delivered – literally!

I've never felt so powerful in my body – in all its messy, wobbly, exhausted glory – as I did in those first few hours and days after our daughter was born.

The advice I give to pregnant friends is to empower yourself with knowledge about what your body is going through – both to help you make informed decisions, but also because it's just a truly amazing feat that you're doing and you should be immensely proud!

Lianne

Fear is an instinct we all have – our ancestors relied on fear responses for their everyday survival. It isn't about ignoring or overlooking your fears, but acknowledging them, challenging them and moving forwards with them. Your fears may have originated from stories that other people have told you about birth, but the good news here is that was their experience, and your pregnancy, baby and birth are unique to you. Perhaps your fears have come from a previous negative experience, your own lived experience. In this case, it is important to remember that this is a different time. Allow yourself to accept that some elements of fear may remain until you have had a different experience, and you'll need to work to ensure that the fear does not control you or take over. Ultimately, the goal is to trust your body more than your fear. Your feelings of trust should outplay any sensations of fear for birth as the two do not complement each other and do not tend to exist in harmony. By allowing trust and positive thoughts to lead, you will simultaneously be suppressing ideas of fear and anxiety.

Let's take a moment to acknowledge any concerns or worries you currently have about your labour and birth. This is a time to be entirely honest with yourself and to use this exercise as a personal, judgement-free space, so do not hold back. As you write down each worry, imagine it being removed from your mind and making space for new positive thoughts that you'll learn in this book. Draw a definite line through your existing concern and then write how you wish to feel about this instead. You may even want to revisit the affirmation exercise above to help you in this and keep these goal feelings in mind as we walk through this book. Each chapter will provide stepping stones, like a bridge between your current worry and your goal.

Current concern	How you wish to feel instead

Every time you find one of the old worries creeping in, remind yourself that allowing this thought to occupy your mind pushes out one of those positive feelings you want to welcome. So pause and recognise the worry and allow yourself to validate and unpick it: *Why do you feel this way? What can you do to address this concern? How can you implement steps to view it in a positive light?* For example: 'What if I need to be induced?' Instead try: 'If I do need to be induced, I will have made that decision for me and my baby with calm confidence, explored all my options and evaluated the evidence. I have the tools and techniques to have a positive induction of labour experience.' If you don't have all the answers right now, that is fine. As you work further through this book they will come, so be sure to refer back to this exercise as and when you need to.

Filtering outside influences

When someone realises you're pregnant or you start looking at pregnancy-related media content, you will be bombarded with birth stories and opinions. For example, that well-meaning colleague who shares their own negative birth story or an article you stumble across online portraying an anti-intervention approach to birth. You may have the confidence to politely ask your colleague to refrain from sharing their story with you while you plan for your own birth, or you may feel the need to vaguely listen, thank them and allow that information to flow into one ear and out of the other. Either method is fine – whichever feels comfortable to you, as long as you do not allow yourself to absorb their negative thoughts.

Be ready to put a filter on anything that feels discouraging by not engaging in certain conversations, unfollowing some social accounts and turning off the TV when needed. You can also create a box in your mind that allows that person's experience to be boxed up – that is their experience, but that does not mean it will be yours. If you do find yourself in a negative birth story conversation, it can also be helpful to ask, 'What would you have done differently?' This then allows the tone of the conversation to switch to them sharing tips with you that may help you in your positive birth preparation.

Viewing pain differently

You have begun setting the foundations for the preparation of your mind ahead of birth through recognising and starting to challenge any fears or anxieties you may have. Now, let's look at how to navigate the term 'pain'. This word can be triggering for some and has such a strong association with labour and birth. If your mind has been conditioned to associate labour with pain and your understanding of pain is something that will trigger negative feelings, then your body will automatically go into a state of fear, anxiety and tension during labour – the fight-or-flight response we met earlier – causing surges in adrenaline and interfering with your oxytocin production, inhibiting your ability to labour physiologically.

But let's also be realistic – you cannot simply avoid the term 'pain' for the whole of your pregnancy, so it is important to understand how pain is different in labour than in other areas of life. The pain felt during labour then becomes a sensation we can embrace in a positive light and not one to feel fearful of. It is also important to recognise that some women may not experience a 'painful' sensation during labour and birth, but others will and this is where being able to calmly and confidently relax into the physiological cycle instead of becoming fearful of these sensations is a valuable tool.

The 'pain' associated with labour and birth is unique. It is:

- Purposeful: for a positive purpose to support the birth of your little one.
- Anticipated: you know these sensations are coming and you have this time during pregnancy to prepare and establish tools and techniques to understand and manage it.
- Intermittent: contractions are like waves – they start, build up, peak and fade away. A little like any HIIT or interval

exercising you may have done before – you work really hard for a minute and then you rest.

- Normal: the sensations are not as a result of something going wrong, they are because your body is doing exactly what it is meant to do and has been designed to do.

The two pain cycles

There are two types of pain: negative, pathological pain and positive, physiological pain. Your body can respond in very different ways depending on which type of pain it perceives to be happening. Physically, labour and birth are the physiological type, and your mindset is your key to showing your body that this is the case. Being able to understand this difference and to manage your labour in the positive pain cycle is important as it ensures your body's key labour hormones can work and that you can experience a more comfortable and smoother labour and birth journey.

Let's compare these two types of pain and how they would work in a labour and birth scenario:

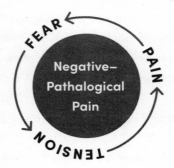

Fight-or-flight response of adrenaline causes blood to go to your limbs rather than your uterus – interfering with contractions and making labour longer/more painful.

The negative, pathological pain cycle

This is the cycle you have experienced before – for example, when you stub your toe or have an injury. In this cycle, your body feels threatened, triggering your fight-or-flight response which releases adrenaline and cortisol, diverting blood away from your uterus, which needs blood to contract in labour. If you can shift this dynamic, and keep a calm and safe mind during labour and birth, your body can behave very differently and this supports the physiological processes of birth.

In this cycle, your body is relaxed and releases powerful endorphins. These are your best friends as endorphins are your body's natural painkillers, and you want to support their production as much as possible. Oxytocin is the dominant hormone in allowing

A relaxed body releases endorphins – a natural pain killer. Oxytocin (love hormones) is also released in larger amounts when we are calm, which aids contractions.

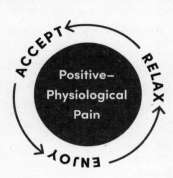

The positive or physiological pain cycle

your uterus to contract, an essential part of labour progress, and is also released in higher amounts when you feel calm and relaxed.

The aim here is for you to focus on breaking the negative cycle of pain and learn to tap into the positive cycle in labour. Facilitating this shift into the positive pain cycle begins with you understanding your body and baby on the journey of birth and building trust and a sense of strength and capability within yourself. The exercise you've done above on recognising your birth worries starts this process off and the chapters that follow will further support you to have a deeper understanding of your incredible female body.

Have you ever watched a mammal other than a human give birth? Check out some videos online of sheep, cats or dogs birthing their babies. Their bodies go through the exact same processes with contractions that we have discussed. But you'll notice something different. Unlike what we see on TV where women appear distressed, these animals stay calm, quiet and move their bodies or pace around instinctively. We know that these animals do feel sensations of pain, but they don't do this when they birth their babies as their minds have not been warped to see birth in the anxiety-provoking way that many human minds have.

By understanding the processes going on in your body, having the knowledge about how incredibly well your body has been preparing to birth your baby and therefore how strong and capable you are, you will be able to view your labour and birth in a positive light.

> *I had always been naturally apprehensive when it came to childbirth. Understanding the science behind why and what my body was doing allowed me to completely trust the process and relax throughout labour and birth.*
>
> Jessica

It is so important to regularly remind yourself of how to view the sensation of pain differently during labour to gradually ease your mind into this new way of thinking about labour and birth.

Remind yourself every single day how strong and capable you are as a woman.

Visualising your baby being born

Visualising the way you wish your birth space to be and how you wish to feel when you welcome your little one into your arms is another really powerful tool to prepare your mind for birth. Close your eyes and take a moment to visualise the moment you welcome your baby into the world in the way you would like it to happen. How do you feel in this moment? Do you feel relaxed? Can you drop your shoulders and relax your jaw a little more? Can you feel their skin against yours? How does that make you feel? Connect to all the positive sensations you feel and allow yourself to revisit these regularly over the coming weeks and months until your baby arrives.

Feelings of relaxation, love and calm are sensations to bring into your life as much as possible as you prepare for birth, whether that is by visualising your little one or by actions that create positive sensations for you, such as walking in nature or having a massage. An aspect of preparing for birth is respecting your body, prioritising your well-being and recognising how capable and strong you are.

While I wouldn't say I am someone who loved the whole labour experience (it was so intense at points), I certainly am in awe of my body and my mental strength. I am seriously proud of myself for staying so centred and focused even during the most challenging parts.

Ali

THE POWER OF POSITIVE BIRTH STORIES

If you are anything like me, reading positive birth stories is an inspiring process, but it is also really informative as you will notice ideas or tips from others' birth experiences that you may wish to bring into your own, especially if there were twists or turns in their birth that you are not sure how you would navigate. Reading others' birth stories can also instil that *'I have got this'* attitude and self-belief in your ability to also have a positive birth experience. Reading the raw strength, courage and capabilities of women birthing their babies gives me goosebumps. There truly is no experience like that of welcoming a new precious life into the world, and those who are willing to share their experiences are an incredible source of support for expectant mums.

Take time to seek out a range of positive birth stories to read or listen to, from all modes of birth – home births, induced births, assisted births, water births, caesarean births – and allow yourself to plan out all these eventualities in your head. I said at the beginning that no one way to birth is superior to another and reading birth stories really helps you to cement this in your mind too. Remember that all births can be positive and empowering.

To make it super easy to seek out a range of experiences, I have gathered together birth stories from some incredible women sharing their journey – scan the QR code on page 6. My own experience is on page 302 too. We really are in this together.

You now know how easily your brain can be influenced, so it is important to safeguard this. As you prepare for your birth, always remember: *'I am ready to birth my baby with calm confidence and am empowered to do so in whatever way is best for me and my baby in our own unique way.'* You can do so much more than you realise and are more capable than you ever dreamed.

The alignment between your mind and body means that some of your physical preparation techniques we will discuss through Part One will also be crucial to your mindset preparation. Your body is incredible and, in the next chapter, we will discuss how it is perfectly designed for birth.

REMEMBER:

- When your mind feels calm, relaxed and safe, your body responds positively to labour.
- The physiological pain cycle presents the opportunity to relax into the sensations and experience a more comfortable labour.
- Affirmations are a really powerful way to help you overcome negative thoughts and create positive changes in your mind.

2

UNDERSTANDING YOUR INCREDIBLE BODY

It is time to feel confident in your body's ability to birth. If you do not realise now how capable you are then by the end of this chapter you will be fastening up your superhero cape.

This is not about teaching you how to give birth – your body already knows how to do that! It is about further convincing your mind that you are capable of doing it too. However, before we can talk about the changes that happen to your body to prepare for birth and explore ways in which you can help the process, we need to first look at your incredible anatomy.

YOUR ANATOMY

The female anatomy has been taboo for far too long and we need to empower women in pregnancy and postpartum by having comfortable conversations about vaginas, vulvas, breasts, and so on. There is going to be a whole load of vagina talk in this chapter – it is such a normal part of my language as a midwife, and it is important that you also feel comfortable talking about your anatomy and learning exactly what is what to really optimise how you understand and can support your body on this journey.

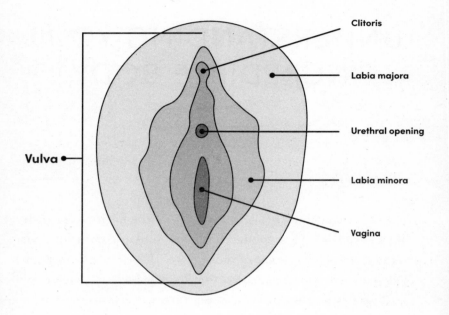

Clitoris

Labia majora

Urethral opening

Labia minora

Vagina

Vulva

VULVA

The EXTERNAL part of the genitalia that includes the labia, clitoris, vaginal opening and the opening to the urethra

VAGINA

The INTERNAL part of the genitalia and the canal that connects the vaginal opening to the cervix.

The vagina

Your vagina is not to be confused (as is so often the case) with the vulva, which is the external genitalia. The vagina is the muscular tube or canal that connects to your cervix (the neck of the womb – see below) and is unique because of its ability to be super-elastic and stretchy to allow your baby to move through it during birth. In fact, it can increase in size by up to 245 per cent during this time. This is why the frankly ludicrous myth that birthing a baby is like pushing a watermelon out of your anus is very inaccurate and can be firmly placed in the rubbish information bin. Your vagina is awesome; it was designed specifically for childbirth. Your vagina can stretch in a way your anus cannot and your baby's head changes in a way a watermelon cannot . . . All hail the vagina!

The cervix

The top of your vagina opens into your cervix (often referred to as the neck of the womb). You may be familiar with this part of your body if you have had a smear test before. Your cervix is a tube, around 3cm long, which sits in front of your baby's head. Your cervix is closed to keep your baby safely housed inside your uterus during pregnancy and it attaches to your uterus (often referred to as the womb) where your baby is growing and developing.

The uterus

Your uterus is pear-shaped and resembles an inflated balloon whereby the balloon is your uterus and the neck of the balloon is your cervix. Your uterus is a thick muscular organ made from three muscle layers:

- The inner layer is made up of circular muscles. They are thick and strong and hold your baby in place during pregnancy.
- The middle layer is a muscular mesh, like a criss-crossing net of muscle fibres, and contains lots of blood vessels and nerves.
- The outer layer is made of strong horizontal muscle fibres.

The variable direction of these different layers of muscle fibres is what gives your uterus its incredible strength and ability to expand up to 1,000 times its original size during pregnancy and to protect your baby so well.

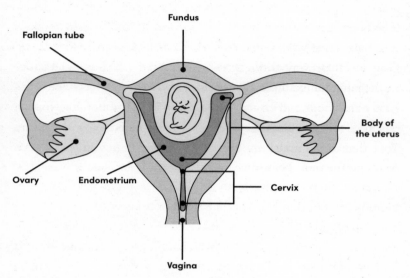

These key parts of your anatomy – your vagina, cervix and uterus – are designed to work harmoniously together during labour and birth. The inner muscle layer of your uterus relaxes, while the outer layer contracts. This pulls the muscles of your cervix upwards into the body of your uterus and causes it to open or dilate. This is the main physical change that happens during the latent and first stage of labour (more on these stages of labour in Part 2).

The uterus is unique to any other muscle in your body. If you contract your bicep muscle, when you relax it, it just goes back to its original state, but your uterus is different. After each contraction of your uterus during labour, the muscle fibres become shorter and thicker, so that, by the time you reach the second stage of labour, when the cervix is fully dilated and your baby is being pushed down the birth canal, you have thick, strong muscle at the top of the uterus to facilitate the next stage.

I have prepared a short video to show you visually how your uterus, cervix and vagina work harmoniously during labour and birth, which you can access via the QR code on page 6.

The pelvis

The other structure that plays a role in birth is your pelvis. Your body and baby must work together during labour to allow your baby to navigate their way through the bony parts of your pelvis. The pubic joint, for example, can increase in diameter by a whole centimetre in labour, which can make a significant difference to how easy it is for your baby to navigate through it. Imagine the difference that would make when you were trying desperately to fit your foot into the most beautiful shoes that were a size too small . . . and of course there are plenty of jokes to be made about that extra centimetre, but that is a topic for another book entirely!

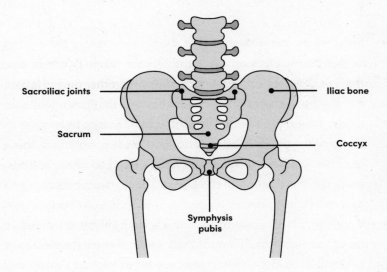

Sacroiliac joints

Sacrum

Iliac bone

Coccyx

Symphysis pubis

How your baby moves through your pelvis

Approximately 96 per cent of babies will present head down at full-term (this is also called cephalic presentation). Their journey begins by passing into the brim of your pelvis when they engage into it. Typically, this happens before labour starts and the angle of your baby's head in relation to the pelvic brim will alter how easy this step is. As your baby moves through your pelvis, they use your pelvic floor muscles to rotate in your mid-pelvis before navigating the outlet to be born. Your pelvis is not a straight line so your baby can't whizz through like a pea shooter. It is more of a twisting and angling journey, with lots of shifting and wriggling, like when you work a ring off your pregnant finger at the end of the day (fluid-retention mums, you get me here).

Your baby's journey through your pelvis looks like this:

- Descent and engagement: baby's head moves down towards the pelvic brim and is classed as 'engaged' once the widest part of their head has negotiated its way deep into the pelvis. Your community midwife will feel for this when palpating your bump.
- Flexion: as baby descends through the pelvis, their head comes into contact with your pelvic floor. When this happens, their neck flexes and they tuck their chin onto their chest to reduce the diameter of their head, making their passage easier.
- Internal rotation: with each contraction, baby's head pushes down onto your pelvic floor and, after each contraction, there is a little rebound which allows baby's head to rotate to complete their navigation of the pelvis. They continue to descend into the vaginal canal.
- Crowning: this happens once the widest diameter of baby's head has successfully negotiated through the narrowest part of your pelvis. Baby's head can be seen at the vulva externally at this stage and birth is imminent.
- Extension: baby's head slips underneath the suprapubic arch (a part of the pelvis that is wider in women than men to allow for a baby to pass through) so the head can extend and be born.

- External rotation and restitution: once baby's head has been born, their shoulders are just reaching the pelvic floor. At this point baby does a little adjustment called restitution to align their head and shoulders before a final rotation and their body is born.

What a journey, right?! But here is the amazing thing: all the way through pregnancy your pelvis has been making changes and adjustments to support this process.

Firstly, the female pelvis is wider than a male pelvis, which makes growing and birthing a baby possible. Then, during pregnancy, higher levels of hormones such as progesterone and relaxin relax your ligaments, loosening joints and increasing the mobility within your pelvis, making your baby's passage easier. The symphysis pubis at the front of your pelvis softens and the sacroiliac joints at the back stretch to make more space for your baby to descend through. The sacrum at the back of your pelvis moves up and out of the way during labour, as does the coccyx (tailbone), and the whole pelvis tilts slightly forwards to enable the birth canal and pelvic outlet to be well-aligned. All of these changes accumulate to help facilitate the passage of your baby that mirrors your natural physiology. Positions you adopt in labour also help to support optimising the diameters of your pelvis – and we'll explore these in Part 2.

I was in complete shock when they handed me our newborn son. It felt like a real out-of-body experience. I honestly couldn't believe what I'd just done. I was in complete awe of my body and my husband for all the unwavering support even when things went 'off plan'. I felt like I was on cloud nine after our birth.

Ali

YOUR BABY'S ADAPTATIONS FOR BIRTH

Your baby is very clever too. Their head and your pelvis are designed to do this incredible little dance together to support the birthing process. Your baby's skull consists of five bones that are not fused, which means they can move as they need to during labour and overlap a little to make your baby's head smaller. Your baby has two fontanelles, which are soft spots covered with a thick, tough membrane. They have a diamond at the front and a triangle at the back and these areas enable the bones to flex during birth and mould the space efficiently, enabling your baby to move through the birth canal during labour. This is called moulding and is often the cause of babies being born with that cone-shaped head (don't worry, this resolves very quickly). If you feel your baby's head when they are born, you will be able to feel the lines where their skull bones meet and the fontanelles – these will fuse completely at around 18 months.

Here is where your baby gets even more impressive, though: the start of labour is initiated by your baby when they are ready by releasing a small amount of a substance from their lungs that signals to your body to start releasing your labour hormones and – voilà – contractions begin.

Your baby has also made very clever adaptations to their physiology in pregnancy in preparation for the big day of their birth. This may be a bit too science-geeky for you, but I am a total birth nerd and find it fascinating how incredibly designed babies are for the journey of birth. Your baby has a much higher haemoglobin (iron) level than you do, which allows them to accumulate much more oxygen, and so meet their oxygen needs even when there isn't as much oxygen readily available during labour. This is a very handy skill as their oxygen supply is temporarily reduced with each contraction. During stressful times in labour, your baby's blood has higher levels of CO_2 and hydrogen and, amazingly, the placenta (the organ you have specially made and grown to act as your baby's personal life support machine while they are inside you) can notice this, then sends out a buffer to mop up these compounds and bring your baby's blood back to a healthier balance. It is like this super-intricate, secret communication between your body, your baby and your placenta. Your baby also has specially stored-away glycogen to use when oxygen levels are lower, too, so they really are expertly designed for this journey of entering the world.

YOUR HORMONES DURING BIRTH

During labour, birth and the immediate postpartum there is a dance happening between your body's hormones, and there are some key players in this process.

Oxytocin

Oxytocin is often called the love hormone because it is produced during sex, orgasm, birth and breastfeeding. It is the lead hormone in birth as it is responsible for stimulating and regulating contractions. The aim in labour is to boost oxytocin and reduce adrenaline to facilitate effective and efficient uterine contractions.

During labour, oxytocin is released by your brain and signals to your uterus to contract; this causes your baby's head to press on to your cervix. Your cervix then sends signals back to your brain to release more oxytocin. The cycle continues, causing your baby to put more pressure on to your cervix, allowing your cervix to dilate and regular, powerful contractions to be produced. Your oxytocin levels rise throughout pregnancy and peak during labour at three to four times higher than your pre-pregnancy levels by the time you give birth. The more oxytocin that is present in your body, the more your body produces, which means the contractions that it generates become more effective and your brain more equipped with all the oxytocin benefits too. Oxytocin helps reduce stress, anxiety and pain during labour by activating your brain's pleasure and reward centres, helping you to feel more relaxed. Synthetic forms of oxytocin given via a drip to induce or augment labour don't have the same effect on a mother as they enter via the bloodstream and cannot cross over into the brain due to the blood–brain barrier, so cannot influence the brain in the same positive way that natural oxytocin does.

Despite being so powerful and influential to your labour, oxytocin is also a shy hormone. If the environment doesn't feel right, the conscious part of your brain is working too hard or your mind perceives a threat, as we explored in the last chapter, oxytocin production reduces, making contractions less effective. This highlights why the environment you create and the way you feel is of such importance in labour as you can hold the key to turning oxytocin on or off. Oxytocin keeps working after your baby is born to help contract your uterus and protect you from haemorrhage.

Adrenaline and noradrenaline

These hormones are responsible for initiating the fight-or-flight response (see page 13) and will be more prominent when you do not feel calm and safe. The fight-or-flight response is important in the context of labour as it can easily be activated, resulting in contractions stopping. When levels of adrenaline and noradrenaline hormones are too high, it can inhibit oxytocin production and, as a result, also cause contractions to slow down or stop.

In the final stages of labour, adrenaline can have the opposite effect and can lead to increased contractions to help you birth your baby quicker.

Endorphins

You will produce your very own, natural, tailor-made pain relief during birth in the form of endorphins. These help relieve pain and can induce a sense of euphoria, especially during labour. The levels of your natural endorphins may be reduced when medical pain relief is used.

However, when endorphin levels are too high during labour, it reduces oxytocin, which can again slow down and reduce the intensity of labour. This may happen if your brain detects that you are too anxious or stressed with the current intensity of labour. Again, this highlights the importance of being able to relax into the process and ensure you maintain the positive, physiological pain cycle, as discussed in Chapter 1. Moderate levels of endorphins are optimal to offer a good level of pain relief without slowing down labour.

Endorphins also allow you to be naturally instinctive during labour and encourage your brain to follow what your powerful maternal instincts are telling you, be that a position to move into or a noise to make. During birth, be mindful and receptive to your natural instincts – it is your body's way of actively helping you out! Endorphin production continues after birth and it is present in breast milk too, which is the reason babies have that happy content look after breastfeeding.

Prolactin

Prolactin is at its most powerful post-birth in preparation to support you with breastfeeding as it is the major hormone responsible for producing breast milk. Your baby suckling at the breast in the early hours and days after birth increases your prolactin levels, which makes your body more responsive to this hormone and, in turn, helps optimise breast milk supply in the long term.

Prolactin also impacts emotional behaviours, helping mothers to prioritise their baby's needs and increasing vigilance and anxiety. This is a protective mechanism designed to ensure a mother meets the physical needs of their baby and can protect them from harm. It is another innate instinct from our ancestors that still lives within us in the modern day.

CONTRACTIONS DURING LABOUR

Put simply, a contraction during labour is the muscle of your uterus contracting and then relaxing in the same way that your leg muscles contract and relax when you exercise. The more you understand exactly what a contraction is and how well your body has been designed to manage contractions, the less intimidating the idea of contractions and labour becomes and the more you can move into the 'I have got this' mindset.

Contractions during labour come in waves: they start, peak and then fade away. On average, contractions last around 60 seconds, so if we look at the wave format, you only have 20 seconds at the peak. Typically, 3–4 contractions happen in a 10-minute period: 1 minute of contraction, 2 minutes of rest, and so on. Over the course of labour, this means that 33 per cent of your time is spent contracting and 67 per cent is spent at rest and recovering. Hopefully, looking at it in this context makes it feel more manageable now? It also means you need to really use that recovery time to rest, regroup with your breathing (I will take you through exactly how to breathe for birth in Chapter 3), hydrate, snack if you want to and protect your labour environment and important hormonal balance.

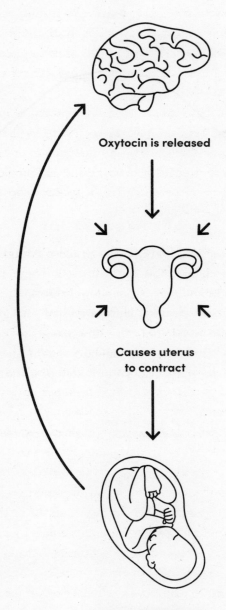

Oxytocin is released

**Causes uterus
to contract**

**Baby's head presses
on cervix**

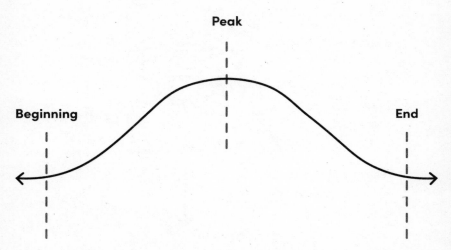

You may notice your body having practice contractions during pregnancy, especially in the third trimester. These are referred to as Braxton Hicks and they happen lower down in the uterus than labour contractions. Braxton Hicks are usually irregular and generally not painful and do not cause any changes to your cervix like the powerful contractions during labour do. They are a very normal part of pregnancy and your body's preparation for labour itself.

'I have the power to do anything I need to accomplish today.'

PAUSE FOR THOUGHT

- How do you feel about your body's ability to birth now you understand your physical and hormonal systems better?
- How do you feel now about contractions?

Self-reflecting like this as we work through this book is really valuable in allowing you to see where you need to focus more, practise affirmations or reread certain elements. It is absolutely fine if you still feel some anxiety or concern over any of these things right now – we are only two chapters in – but, as we continue, keep in mind how your thoughts change and welcome the positive charge that will creep in.

Round of applause to you Mumma – it looks like your body and baby have got everything you need on this birth journey. Having this knowledge about your own body, and the way you and your baby are so well-designed for contractions, labour and birth, means you can begin to build your self-confidence in this process and better understand how our next two chapters will support you and your baby on this journey.

The female body in birth and the way your body adapts, changes and prepares is incredible, and you deserve to know exactly what is happening during your birth. When you understand this, you can better recognise how to help optimise your physiology, so this underlying knowledge is power.

Next, we will unlock the breathing practices that will support you through your birth and beyond.

REMEMBER:

- Your body was designed to birth your baby and, even without you knowing, it has been preparing for this since the start of your pregnancy.
- Your labour hormones are on your side and there to help you out. Recognise their power and keep their balance in check.
- Contractions are powerful and not something to fear – they are a sign that your body and baby are working together harmoniously.

3

UNLOCKING BREATHING TOOLS FOR BIRTH AND BEYOND

In the previous two chapters, we looked at why keeping calm and relaxed in labour is so important, and now we'll explore some of the tools you need to help this happen. I encourage you to open your mind as you work through this chapter because, on the surface, it may seem too simple, perhaps a little 'woo-woo' and not your thing at all. I get you, because that was once me, but the truth is, the advice in this chapter can make a huge difference, ensuring your birth feels manageable and utterly wonderful.

I have supported so many birthing women as a midwife and one recurring theme I see is just how influential the breath is. If you can control your breathing during contractions, then your labour will become much calmer. Throughout your pregnancy, practise your breathing and know that the breathing techniques we'll explore in this chapter can be used during birth (for both a vaginal and caesarean birth), through vaginal examinations or, in fact, any moment that feels overwhelming.

Next, I am going to walk you through the two different breaths and how and when to practise them.

Breathwork is an immensely powerful and
transformative tool at your disposal.

UPWARDS AND DOWNWARDS BREATHING

Labour can be divided into two parts for the purpose of breathing:

1. Upwards labour: the latent (earliest, warm-up stage) and first
   phase (the majority of the time spent in labour sits in the
   first stage). We can call this upwards labour because the work
   your body is doing is moving in an upwards direction. Your
   cervix is being pulled upwards into the sides of your uterus to
   dilate or open it.
2. Downwards labour: the second stage of labour (the final, pushing phase). In this stage, the direction is downwards because
   your baby is travelling down the birth canal to be born.

In Chapter 8 I will explain exactly what happens in each of these
stages of labour, how they are defined and how you can recognise
their differences. For now, with these two stages in mind, you want
to breathe in the direction of travel for your body. So, this means
breathing upwards in the upwards stages and downwards in the
downwards stage.

We have talked about how incredibly connected our minds
and bodies are and, as we breathe in a direction, we can support
our breath with an accompanying visualisation. As you breathe
upwards, you can think upwards. And as you breathe downwards, you
can think downwards as your baby is directed downwards through
the birth canal to be welcomed earthside.

So, how do you breathe or think in a 'direction'?

'Breathe in calm, breathe out tension.'

The upwards breath

The upwards breath helps you feel calm and relaxed in all aspects of your life, not just during labour, and it can be really helpful, especially in the fourth trimester (the 12-week period after you've had your baby). This breath is simple and effective in slowing down your heart rate, and encouraging your body and mind to relax – and the more relaxed you are, the easier labour and birth will be.

The key with breathing for birth is practice, so that it slots naturally into place when contractions start, and you aren't trying to learn something new while also navigating labour. Take some time between now and the arrival of your baby to practise this breathing technique. Try to aim for five minutes each day, but of course more if you can. I find it really helpful to work through a cycle of five upwards breaths first thing in the morning and whenever something crops up that makes me feel like my stress and anxiety sensors are on high alert. It is a great technique that you can do anywhere that has a quick impact on calming down your nervous system, and the more you can practise using it the more effective it will feel during birth.

I recall so vividly the first time the upwards breath kicked in for me during labour – I was in my living room, swaying from side to side, and I felt an incredibly powerful sense of control by instinctively tapping into my breathing and feeling an instant softening of any tension through my pelvis.

How to do it

Take a comfortably long breath in through your nose (or mouth if you are planning on using gas and air in labour – see Chapter 13 for more on this). This may be between four and six seconds, depending on your lung capacity – don't put too much emphasis on a specific number, just make sure it is a comfortable length. Follow your inhale with a longer exhalation through your mouth of six to eight seconds.

It is that simple! Repeating this exercise four or five times will support you through a whole contraction.

By taking that slow, extended exhale, you tell your mind and body that you're calm and safe. This then signals to your body to stop producing adrenaline so that your body is able to produce plenty of the wonderful oxytocin needed to support your labour and birth process, as we discussed in Chapter 2.

You can build on this breathing technique by connecting it with an upwards visualisation. Close your eyes and imagine a coloured balloon deflated in your pelvic area. As you inhale, that balloon inflates and fills your abdomen. As you exhale, it floats out of your abdomen and off up, up, up into the sky. You can use any upwards-motion object you like, so feel free to play around with ideas.

From my past experiences I was not looking forward to labour. The breathing techniques I learned made the most amazing difference for me. I used the visualisations to relax into a rhythm during labour and my midwife said it was 'peaceful to watch' because I went to a truly chilled mental space. I didn't even register the passing of time and it was over halfway through labour before I had any pain relief (even gas and air).

Clare

The downwards breath

With downwards breathing, you still want to feel relaxed, but you also need to be more active and purposeful with your breath to support the movement of your baby. Imagine trying to blow out a candle using a slow exhale compared to a purposeful blow – the purposeful active breath is going to be much more effective.

As your body moves into this second, downwards stage of labour, many women feel an urge to bear down or push in an involuntary and instinctive way, like when you really need a poo. As you feel your body begin to push down, you can use your breath to help your baby navigate their way down. If this happens, do not fear it, go with it and trust the process, allowing yourself to push or breathe in the way that feels right, keeping in mind the downwards nature in this stage. This involuntary urge to push is called the 'Ferguson reflex' and is initiated by your baby's head moving down and stimulating the stretch receptors in the posterior wall of your vagina. When this happens, it signals to your brain to release even more oxytocin, which in turn further initiates the Ferguson reflex and leads to an uncontrollable feeling of needing to push. This is a fantastic example of your body knowing instinctively what it needs to do, and it is important not to fight this sensation, but recognise how normal and wonderfully powerful the process is; trust in it and go with it.

A key message here is to follow your instincts and, if your body takes over this powerful stage with involuntary pushing down, go with it. While you can use the downwards breath to support the process, don't fight the bearing down urge in favour of the breath, because whatever your body is instinctively feeling at this stage is right.

How to do it

When your contraction builds, take a sharp, quick, deep breath inwards and then, as you exhale, send that energy down towards your bottom with action and purpose. If you place your hands on your abdomen, you will feel your muscles engage as you exhale. In between contractions, relax and resume your normal breathing until the next one begins to build.

The downwards breath may be a little trickier to feel confident with, but thankfully there is an ideal time to practise . . . you guessed it, when you go for a poo! This is honestly the most similar sensation to your baby being birthed. Avoid straining and rushing, and instead use your downwards breath. It takes a bit of practice and perseverance at first, but it is also a much gentler way to poop for your pelvic floor and prevents excessive pressure and strain through these muscles, which over time can cause some damage to your pelvic floor. Pooping with the downwards breath is a great technique for life, but doubles up as birth preparation in pregnancy too.

If you have daily bowel habits then using the downwards breath allows for easy daily practice. If you're not so regular at pooping then do not worry – it is still best to use your toilet time to practise this breath, so just wait until you do need to poo. Another moment when the downwards breath can be practised is if you choose to perform perineal massage during the final weeks of your pregnancy. This is a gentle massage of the muscles and skin between your vagina and anus, and I will guide you through everything you need to know about this technique in Chapter 14.

With the downwards breath, many women like to visualise exactly what they are doing, for example, moving your baby down the birth canal, with your baby getting closer and closer as each contraction passes.

Breathing techniques helped me so much in labour. I'd been practising them throughout my pregnancy when pooping. I went into labour at 1am and didn't have my little girl until 1.23am the following day. My labour stagnated once in hospital and the last two centimetres were long! And ended in forceps. But I felt totally prepared and full of energy and put that down to breathing, managing my energy by being calm and some really good snacks. Since having my baby I still use the breathing techniques when I'm in a stressful situation or have injured myself – it's really a great technique just to regulate yourself.

Niomi

VALSALVA MANOEUVRE

You may have seen or heard of this technique for pushing during the final stage of labour. The Valsalva manoeuvre is when you are asked to take a deep breath in, hold your breath and push downwards with a contraction until you can't hold your breath anymore. Then breathe in again quickly and do the same. Evidence has challenged this mode of pushing as it has been linked with a reduction in oxygen supply to baby, exhaustion in mothers and increased vaginal tearing. An alternative method of pushing through the use of downwards breathing and spontaneous, involuntary pushing leads to better release of oxytocin, resulting in more effective contractions, better movement of your baby through your pelvis and quicker labour.

As with everything in pregnancy and birth, it is not black and white, though – there is a balance to be achieved and variables may crop up, for example, some women with an epidural may not be aware of their contractions or have any sensation, which can prevent them feeling this involuntary pushing urge and so more coached pushing may be necessary. This was true in my own birthing experience – I utilised my body's instinctive urges to bear down and used the downwards breath, but then my baby's heart rate showed some changes and, at that stage, I made an informed decision to move to a more directed pushing-down method to speed up his birth. The reason I want to share this experience with you is to highlight how there is flexibility in the way you push and you may find that a mixed method works best. Your midwife will be there to guide you on this.

RELAX YOUR JAW TO SOFTEN YOUR PELVIC FLOOR

When you are practising your breathing techniques, try to totally relax your jaw and let it go all floppy and loose. When you do this, notice how your shoulders, abdomen and pelvic floor also relax. This is because these parts of our body are all connected, so when you relax your jaw, you relax everything else, which is so important during labour. Your birth partner can watch out for you tensing up here and remind you to relax and reconnect with your breath. Remember, by relaxing much of your body, including your pelvis and pelvic floor, you are helping your labour hormones do their thing in the beautiful way they are designed to. If you do find tension building in your jaw and shoulders during labour, it can be helpful to do some gentle swaying side to side or dance if you want to – just focus on loosening everything up and letting it all go. Trust in the process and capability of your body, relax and go along with the ride. A relaxed body is a body that will be able to dance with the powerful hormones needed for labour to progress and to stay distant from the negative pain cycle of tension and fear.

PAUSE FOR THOUGHT

When are you going to fit in your daily breathing practice? First thing in the morning? When you get into bed at night? During your bath? Find your time and commit to it – your birthing self will be so grateful that you did.

Your breathing practice is a powerhouse to help you achieve your positive birth, but there are other tools and techniques I want to equip you with on this journey to help you too. In the next chapter, we will be discussing how to prepare physically for your birth.

REMEMBER:

- Practise the upwards breath daily in pregnancy. Four to five breaths is a whole contraction.
- Practise the downwards breath when you go for a poo – it is a short, sharp and purposeful breath.
- Your instincts in birth are powerful – give yourself the space to recognise and respond to them.

4

PREPARING PHYSICALLY FOR YOUR BIRTH

Now you have an understanding of your body and how your mindset, hormones and breathwork interact and influence each other, I am going to take you through the physical ways you can prepare for birth.

Throughout this chapter, I will be equipping you with must-know tools for a calmer birth, such as how you can use exercise to influence your birth, how to support your pelvic floor and, one of my favourite topics, helping your baby be in the best position for a smoother labour and birth. I will also talk you through nutritional support as well as some of the facts around things you can try to naturally encourage labour in late pregnancy.

MOVING YOUR BODY FOR A BETTER BIRTH

It is useful to think of the physical side of birth a bit like that of a marathon. Picture a marathon runner: before they take on the challenge of a marathon, they have months to prepare their minds and bodies for it. Birth (and motherhood) is your marathon, and pregnancy is your opportunity to train your body for the demands of possibly the biggest and most important endurance event of your life. The good news is, I am not prescribing you 20+ miles of running, but I am going to strongly advise you to do some physical activity specific to the demands of pregnancy and birth.

Pregnancy is a fantastic opportunity to positively influence the health of yourself and your growing baby. By exercising in pregnancy, you can reduce the chance of pregnancy and birth complications and aid a smoother postpartum recovery. A minimum of 150 minutes of moderate-intensity exercise per week is currently recommended during pregnancy, and pregnant women are encouraged to perform muscle-strengthening activities twice a week as part of this. Please be reassured that this does not mean you have to hit the gym and start pumping iron (unless of course you wish to!), but when your baby is born you will be lifting and carrying them (essentially an ever-growing dumbbell) in all sorts of positions, lugging prams around (the average weight of a pram is 15kg), and you are currently doing squats every time you get on and off the toilet or sofa. You need to be able to perform these everyday movements and tasks without injury. And labour, of course, is a physically exerting challenge; your cardiovascular system will be working as well as your muscle strength and flexibility to move between the best positions for you and your baby, so your body needs to be physically prepared for this event.

Exercise is also a fantastic tool to help reinforce that sense of strength and self-confidence ahead of birth. You should be empowered to exercise during pregnancy and supported to feel powerful, capable and strong along the way, regardless of your ability or current fitness level. There are a few (very few) conditions where your midwife or obstetrician (a doctor who specialises in pregnancy, birth and the early postnatal period) will advise against physical activity, but, for the vast majority, it is hugely beneficial with reduced risk of developing gestational diabetes, high blood pressure, poor sleep and depression symptoms to name a few benefits.

If you have not exercised previously that is OK – this is a great time to start (yes, you can start in pregnancy), but keep it gradual and consider working with a pregnancy exercise specialist if you can.

There is so much movement you can safely do in pregnancy and just a few limitations: avoid high-altitude sports, sports with a high risk of contact such as kick-boxing and rugby, scuba diving or exercising in extreme heat. It is also recommended to avoid or adapt exercises where you lie flat on your back for prolonged periods, elevating your shoulders on a glute bridge exercise for example, as your baby bump weight presses on your main blood vessel responsible for bringing blood back to your heart, and this may make you feel faint. If you enjoy yoga or Pilates, these are great exercises to continue in pregnancy, but you may find a pregnancy-specific class a better option as it will accommodate these adaptations for you.

Not sure where to start? Scan the QR code on page 6 and join me with a do-anywhere pregnancy-safe workout.

The benefits of exercising during pregnancy should not be underestimated, with better recovery post-birth being a huge motivating factor. It's empowering too, and reminds you of just how strong you are and what you are capable of! Don't shy away from keeping active during pregnancy; after all, you are preparing your body for birth and will feel so much better prepared knowing you've done everything you can to build your stamina and endurance.

Lucy

BETTER POSTURE FOR A MORE COMFORTABLE PREGNANCY

You are more susceptible to pelvic, back and hip pain in pregnancy because of changing hormones, weight gain, pelvic floor lengthening, diastasis recti (see page 289) and a postural shift as your bump grows. Keeping your body strong and active and being aware of keeping your pelvis aligned in a neutral position (without too much of a forward lean and curving back as your bump grows) are great and simple ways to help to avoid, manage and improve this.

The diagram on page 60 shows the common posture women adopt in pregnancy that often results in pain through the back, hips and pelvis compared to a more aligned, neutral stance (see page 61) where your back and pelvis are better supported.

HELPING YOUR BABY INTO THE BEST POSITION FOR BIRTH

If I could gift you one thing when you go into labour, it would be this: for your baby to be in an optimal position. If your baby is in an optimal position you are more likely to have a smoother, quicker labour with a reduced chance of severe perineal tears, as well as interventions such as instrumental birth and a reduced chance of an emergency caesarean birth. And this is why I wish I had a magic wand for everyone ahead of birth. While I am still working on that, I am going to share with you something equally as powerful: understanding and knowledge so that you can actively encourage your baby into a great position for birth.

Optimising positioning is about encouraging your baby into one of the easier positions for them to navigate your pelvis and birth canal. Your baby may change position for many different reasons, such as tightness or excessive laxity in the soft tissues supporting your uterus, pelvis and abdomen, the location of your placenta, the shape of your uterus or pelvis and the positions you move in. Some of these reasons are out of your control, which means, for some mums, despite trying everything I recommend, their baby still may not be in a favourable position. However, for most, you *can* influence your baby's position and therefore your birth.

So, what are you trying to achieve? For your baby to be head down, facing your spine with their back towards the front of your tummy:

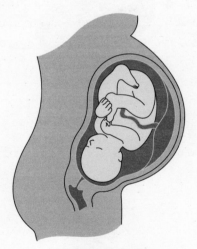

Occiput-anterior

This is called the occiput-anterior or OA position, and the reason this position is beneficial is because it provides the easiest passage through your pelvis for your baby. The part of their head navigating your pelvis is smaller, they can tuck their chin well, curve their back easier and place even pressure on to your cervix, which helps it to dilate without complications like swelling.

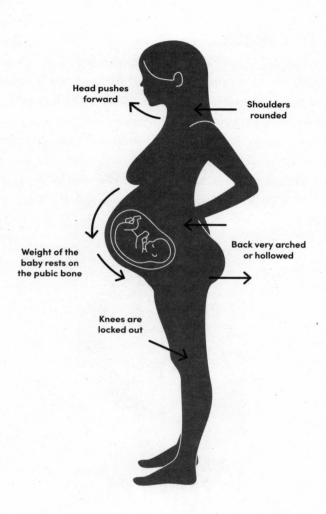

Head pushes forward

Shoulders rounded

Weight of the baby rests on the pubic bone

Back very arched or hollowed

Knees are locked out

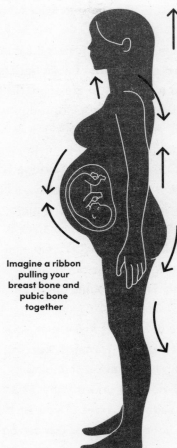

Pull the back of your head up to the ceiling

Pull just your shoulders back and down, not your chest

Stack your pelvis under your rib cage and flatten your lower back by tucking in your tail bone

Imagine a ribbon pulling your breast bone and pubic bone together

Soften your knees slightly

There are lots of variations on positions babies may present in, as well as different pelvis shapes that may lead to a baby preferring one position over another. Work can be done to help optimise this in labour itself, but it is best if you can start your labour already there.

The positions you adopt day to day have a huge influence on this in the later weeks of pregnancy. Your baby's back is the heaviest part of their body, and it moves with gravity to the lowest side of your tummy. This means that if you spend your days slouched back on the sofa, sitting in a car or at an office desk, your baby's back will be encouraged to move towards your spine, resulting in an occiput-posterior, or OP, position. This position is associated with longer labours, higher rates of exhaustion, back pain in labour and increased levels of medical intervention. So, where possible, we want to move your baby so their back is facing forwards (OA) rather than facing your back (OP). Changing positions so that you are in more upright and forward-leaning postures is a great tool to encourage this. Here are some tips to try out:

- When on a chair, have your knees lower than your pelvis and your upper body tilted slightly forwards, keeping your back nice and straight and trying to avoid slumping.
- For a resting seated position you can try to sit with your elbows resting on a surface in front of you such as a desk, leaning forwards with your knees apart. This can be done with a chair, but also works really well with a birthing ball.
- Kneeling, forward-leaning positions are also great. Having wider knees allows space for your bump and if you wish you can rest your arms and forehead on a chair, sofa or birthing ball in front of you. This is a great position for labour too and one I used in my own labour quite instinctively.
- All-fours positions such as child's pose, cat cow or wiggling your hips back and forth or side to side can help.

- Try squats and lunges to help your baby navigate the twists and turns of the pelvis and allow gravity to help your baby get nice and low down.
- Stretch out your pelvis and the surrounding muscles to prevent any restrictions and tightness.
- When lying down, try to lie on your left with a peanut ball or pillows between your knees. A peanut ball has a dent in the middle and allows you to lie down without needing to lie flat on a bed in a semi-recumbent position, which is really unhelpful for labour. The peanut ball acts as a support for your top leg to keep your pelvis in an open position so that your baby can rotate into a great position for birth, even while you're lying down resting or sleeping.
- Birthing balls make great alternatives to sofas and chairs. A birthing ball is a big round ball you may have seen in a gym setting before. Having the right-size ball is important for it to be effective – when sat on it, your hips should be in line with your knees or 5–8cm higher than your knees. A 65-cm ball is great for most women, but if you are taller than 5ft 8in you will benefit from a 75-cm ball. (I would recommend purchasing a ball to use at home in the later stages of pregnancy and checking with your local unit if they have access to birthing balls and peanut balls you can use.)
- Embrace daily activity such as walking or swimming to keep you mobile.

Your body and baby will thank you for trying to encourage optimal positioning and it often helps with pregnancy aches and pains too.

'My baby gives me the strength to do anything.'

YOUR PELVIC FLOOR HEALTH

I cannot provide you with a birth preparation book without discussing the pelvic floor and female pelvic health with you. It is a topic fundamental to your well-being as a woman, today and for your future, but also one that is sadly underdiscussed and often found in the taboo box with a firmly shut lid.

One of the reasons it is so important we cover this is because pelvic floor problems are very common, and pregnancy and birth weaken your pelvic floor, which means you may be more likely to experience pelvic floor dysfunction symptoms if you aren't aware of pelvic health (see page 68).

The pelvic floor is a 'sling' of muscles, a bit like a hammock, that runs between your pubic bone in the front and your tailbone at the back. It supports your abdominal organs including your uterus, bowel, bladder and vagina. Your pelvic floor has a really important job to perform as, when functioning correctly, it prevents prolapse (when one or more of these organs slip down from their normal position and bulge into the vagina); leaking of urine, wind or poo; pelvic pain; and painful sex, among other things.

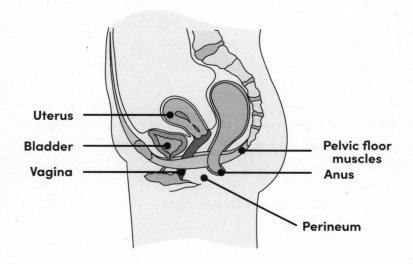

64

When it comes to pregnancy, your pelvic floor muscles are lengthened, stretched and weakened by hormones such as relaxin and progesterone. In addition to this, you also have a fair amount of extra weight on your pelvic floor from the weight of your baby, placenta, extra blood volume, enlarged uterus, and so on. So, extra weight is added on to an already weakened muscle. All of this means that your pelvic floor muscle becomes weakened through pregnancy and there may then also be injury to it during birth. This is why I recommend giving it some extra TLC at this time in your life.

During a vaginal birth, your baby makes contact with your pelvic floor and uses it to flex their neck and tuck their chin on to their chest, reducing the diameter of their head and therefore making their passage easier. Your pelvic floor needs to be strong enough to facilitate this action, but not too tight and rigid or 'overactive' that it inhibits it. Correctly performing pelvic floor exercises helps ensure your pelvic floor is functioning well.

Pelvic floor exercises

So, what are pelvic floor exercises and how do you do them? You may be familiar with the term 'Kegels' – this is simply a name for contracting your pelvic floor. Sit comfortably and relaxed. If this is brand new to you, it is easier to start lying down on your back and then progress to sitting, then standing. If you are heavily pregnant and haven't done these exercises before, it may feel more challenging than in the earlier weeks, but there is still great benefit from doing them, so persevere and it will really help with your post-birth recovery.

Imagine you are squeezing your back passage like you are holding in wind. Then, at the same time, imagine squeezing to lift your vagina. Voilà – that is you contracting your pelvic floor. It can be helpful to use a mirror and see if you notice a slight lift of your perineum (the area between your vaginal opening and anus) or vulva when you engage your pelvic floor. You may also want to place one finger gently inside your vagina and feel a lift or squeeze against your finger.

It's a much smaller and more subtle movement than we imagine, especially in comparison to, say, when we contract a large muscle like our bicep. To learn the movement and generate the best muscle contraction you can it is best to perform these while focusing on doing them, then, over time, as you become more confident, you will find you can do them almost anywhere. At first, it can feel challenging, but, with time and practice, it gets easier and easier until, when you go to cough, your pelvic floor instantly contracts to support you.

Along with contracting, you also need to know how to relax the muscle. Just as when you work your bicep you contract and relax, the same goes for your pelvic floor. A pelvic floor that is too tight is as equally dysfunctional as a pelvic floor that is too weak, so make sure, as you come out of a squeeze, you really allow everything to soften – your jaw, pelvic floor and hips should be free of tension in between squeezes.

When doing pelvic floor exercises, try to remain relaxed – you should be able to breathe and even talk as normal, and your shoulders, buttocks, abdomen and thighs shouldn't be tensing when you squeeze.

To really understand how to do your pelvic floor exercises it is useful to know that your pelvic floor muscle, just like any other muscle in your body, has two types of fibre: slow and fast twitch. The slow twitch fibres are responsible for keeping your pelvic floor holding up your abdominal organs and preventing leaking as you go about your normal everyday activities. Your fast twitch fibres need to kick in when you do things like cough, sneeze, laugh or jump to prevent leakage or incontinence issues. Both types of muscle fibre need to be functioning well for your pelvic floor to be healthy, and therefore, when performing pelvic floor exercises, it is important to work both types of muscle fibre.

Below is a simple routine to follow to ensure you are working both your slow and fast twitch muscle fibres in your pelvic floor. Try to perform this little pelvic floor workout two to three times daily. You could start trying when you're lying in bed in the morning or on the sofa or in bed in the evening. Spacing them out is a good idea to prevent your pelvic floor getting too tired, also known as pelvic floor DOMS (delayed onset muscle soreness).

To work the slow twitch fibres, try to do 10 long squeezes and relaxes. The aim is to hold each long squeeze for 10 seconds. If this is too tricky, try holding for 4–5 seconds and gradually increase it. Then relax for an equal amount of time.

After your set of 10 long squeezes, try to do 10 quick, fast, snappy 1-second squeezes with a 2-second relaxation to work those fast twitch muscle fibres.

Ten of each won't take you more than three minutes and, ideally, you should perform this mini routine two to three times a day from as soon as you find out you're pregnant, throughout your pregnancy and postpartum. This will take you less than ten minutes in total to complete.

When you start pelvic floor exercises, try to really focus on the technique and ensure that you aren't recruiting your bottom, leg or tummy muscles instead. The goal is to generate a really great muscle contraction from within the pelvic floor – and with no other muscle helping you. In time, the great thing is you can do them while doing everyday tasks like watching TV, sitting at traffic lights, brushing your teeth or even waiting for the kettle to boil.

What many women aren't aware of is that pelvic floor exercises should actually be performed for life, in the same way you maintain your oral health by brushing your teeth daily, but they are of extra importance in pregnancy and postpartum. In fact, insider tip: I have a Post-it note on my bathroom mirror as a pelvic floor reminder each morning. Create this as a habit in your pregnancy that you can then continue postpartum. Your pelvic floor exercises are the same post-birth as in pregnancy, so having this nailed will be one less thing to have to learn with a newborn in tow.

Pelvic floor dysfunction

We have been done a huge injustice as women when things such as urine leakage when we go for a run or jump on a trampoline are normalised. The first myth to bust is that this is common, yes, but it is not normal – it is a sign of pelvic floor dysfunction and is not something you should ever simply accept or put up with. Pelvic floor problems are very common, and pregnancy and birth weaken your pelvic floor, which means you may be more likely to experience pelvic floor dysfunction symptoms if you aren't aware of pelvic health. Over 60 per cent of women in the UK are currently experiencing symptoms of a dysfunctional pelvic floor, including leaking of urine, wind or poo; fear of leaking; pelvic and lower back pain; pain when having sex; and recurrent urinary tract infections. Fifty per cent of postpartum women are currently living with a pelvic organ prolapse and women may feel a heaviness, dragging or bulging symptom in the vagina. This is why learning about your pelvic floor and how you can proactively try to support it during times of pregnancy and birth is so beneficial for you. With an understanding of your pelvic floor, you can support your body through this time in your life and help to minimise the chance of any complications.

If you are currently experiencing any symptoms of pelvic floor dysfunction, such as leaking urine, wind or poo, a feeling of heaviness or dragging in your pelvic or vaginal region, urgency to pass urine, lower back or pelvic pain and pain during intercourse, referral to a pelvic health physiotherapist is essential. This can be done in pregnancy and does not need to wait until after birth.

Here are three top tips for your pelvic floor during pregnancy by pelvic health specialist physiotherapist and author of *Why Did No One Tell Me?*, Emma Brockwell, aka @physiomumuk:

1. *Do your pelvic floor exercises daily during pregnancy. Rest assured, we have strong evidence that you won't be wasting your time if you do this. The science shows that pelvic floor exercises can help resolve, reduce and even prevent symptoms of pelvic floor dysfunction! Did you know that pregnant, continent women who exercise the pelvic floor muscles are 62 per cent less likely to experience urinary incontinence in late pregnancy and have a 29 per cent lower risk of urinary incontinence three to six months postpartum? A great win that doesn't take a lot of time!*

2. *Avoid constipation! Constipation is common during pregnancy, but it often leads to straining on the toilet, which places pressure on your pelvic floor and pelvic organs, and this can sometimes lead to pelvic floor dysfunction. To overcome constipation, moving frequently, drinking often and eating a healthy diet can be hugely beneficial. When you need to open your bowels, avoid straining and place a stool under your feet when sitting on the toilet (this helps your pelvic floor relax and makes pooing easier). If these tricks alone aren't enough, please speak to your GP and discuss the use of laxatives, as these can be super effective.*

3. *Visit a pelvic health physiotherapist. I highly recommend all women do this postpartum, but I also encourage you to do so during your pregnancy. Every woman is an individual and every pregnancy is different. A pelvic health physiotherapist will carry out a global pelvic health/musculoskeletal assessment (and ideally include an abdominal and pelvic floor muscle screening). From this, they will provide you with an individualised approach to your physical and pelvic health. We even help you prepare for childbirth! The aim – a proactive approach to your pregnancy and postpartum recovery.*

NOURISHING YOUR BODY AND BABY FOR BIRTH

During pregnancy your stored nutrients and diet are the sole nutrition sources for your baby, and good nutrition in pregnancy has been shown to reduce the chance of adulthood diseases for your baby such as diabetes and high blood pressure.

The exciting thing is that, as you read this, you are in this window of immense opportunity. Regardless of how far into your pregnancy you are, you can nourish yourself and your baby in a way that will have a great positive impact on your growing baby and your mental and physical health as you prepare for birth and being a new parent.

Prioritising your nutrition throughout pregnancy is a brilliant way to boost your mental health and well-being, and the foods you eat will also allow your body to be in the best place to be energised to manage labour, birth, recovery and the demands of motherhood.

Here is some expert advice from Rhiannon Lambert, aka @rhitrition, registered nutritionist and *Sunday Times* bestselling author of *The Science of Nutrition*:

Pregnancy can be a very difficult time for many women. Not everyone will find it easy. Symptoms can range from a lack of appetite due to various different hormonal changes, nausea, aversion to food, reflux and general fatigue, making smart nutritional choices even harder. Some women may even suffer from hyperemesis gravidarum – an extreme and persistent condition of nausea and vomiting throughout pregnancy. In those particular cases, you should seek support from your GP or health professional, as additional fluids and supplementation may be required due to dehydration, weight loss and electrolyte imbalances.

In general, women should aim to follow a Mediterranean-style diet, with the core focus being on fresh, seasonal produce, plant-based eating and healthy unsaturated fats (especially from olive oil). Vegetables, legumes (beans and lentils), whole grains and nuts should form the bulk of meals, with moderate animal protein coming from oily fish and poultry.

All women should be aware that they need to be taking a daily 10mcg vitamin D supplement, as deficiency during pregnancy has been linked to an increased risk of a child developing ADHD and a reduction in IQ and language abilities. Folic acid should also be supplemented during preconception and early pregnancy at a daily dose of 400mcg, to help the body make healthy blood cells, and enable the embryo's brain, skull and spinal cord to develop properly (avoiding neural tube defects, such as spina bifida).

Within my own clinic, I personally recommend women take a multi-vitamin because it can be hard to achieve some nutritional requirements throughout pregnancy. Iron (especially in the third trimester) is also vital during pregnancy, as up to 50 per cent of pregnant women are iron-deficient, which may cause irreversible neural issues in the foetus. Women with gestational diabetes are especially at risk. Foods such as shellfish, broccoli, tofu, nuts, beans and dried fruit are all good sources.

The Food Standards Agency warns that too much caffeine can result in miscarriage or a low birth weight. The NHS advises pregnant women to drink no more than two cups of regular coffee, or less than 200mg caffeine, per day. It is also important to note that other foods such as chocolate and medications also contain caffeine, so it would be easy to exceed the recommended limit without realising.

Leading child health experts worldwide agree that care given from conception to a child's second birthday (the first 1,000 days) has more influence on a child's future than at any other time in their life, and this includes what the mother's diet looks like. There has been a lot of research into the nutrition a baby receives from its mother inside the womb and through breast milk. Babies start to develop their taste preferences for certain flavours within the womb, delivered by amniotic fluid that surrounds them and via breastfeeding. What we expose a baby to when they are inside the womb may predict their food preferences later in life. For example, if you as the mother are eating carrots, there is data that shows that, when the baby is weaning, they have a preference for carrots.

Just to reassure you, the baby is going to get all the nutrients that it needs from you. But it's you who is going to be left short at the end of the day, with a lack of energy and struggling to cope. The good news is that as long as you avoid certain risky foods and drinks, enjoy a generally healthy diet and lifestyle, and pay attention to particular nutrients that are key to a baby's development such as vitamin D, iron and folic acid, you should be on the right track.

GOOD SOURCES OF IRON

- meat
- pulses (beans, peas and lentils)
- fresh green leafy vegetables, such as cabbage, spinach, watercress, parsley and spring onions
- seeds, such as sunflower or sesame seeds
- dried prunes, raisins, figs and apricots
- fish such as grilled mackerel and tinned tuna
- wholegrains, such as brown rice
- nuts, such as almonds, hazelnuts and Brazil nuts

Consuming fruits and vegetables containing vitamin C with iron-rich foods will also help your body to absorb the iron you eat. Try to avoid drinking tea and coffee with an iron-rich meal, because caffeine and milk can stop iron being absorbed into your body.

When it comes to labour itself, food should be at the top of your birth bag (see page 90). Your stomach is unlikely to tolerate a full meal during labour, but will benefit from bits of energy, especially if your labour is on the longer side.

Hydration is also important to think about in labour and birth. While we want to steer clear of dehydration, there is more recent guidance and evidence around why it is also important not to drink excessively during labour and birth. Drinking too much in labour can lead to a condition called hyponatraemia, which means low blood sodium (salt) levels, which can be dangerous for mums and babies. In pregnancy and labour you are at higher risk of hyponatraemia because of your increased blood volume which, like adding water to squash, dilutes the squash (your salt levels). Because you and your baby share the same blood circulation, hyponatraemia in a mother can impact the baby too and cause injury to the brain. A recent study showed that of women who drank over 2,500ml in labour, 26 per cent had hyponatraemia compared to less than 1 per cent in those who had 1,000ml. This explains why your midwife will be keeping an eye on how much you are drinking and peeing during labour. A sensible approach is to sip fluids throughout, to thirst, using an easy-to-drink bottle or straw which your birth partner can support you with. Writing this takes me back to my own birth where I was switching between the birthing pool and the loo between contractions, and each time before I hopped back into the pool, my husband would produce half a jelly baby and a water bottle for a quick nibble, sip and hydrate, similar to a pit stop on any endurance race. Your midwife may also test your urine during labour for the presence of ketones which can suggest dehydration, especially if you are sweating or vomiting as this will cause you to lose fluid.

NATURAL WAYS TO ENCOURAGE LABOUR

The truth is that so many factors may affect when you may go into labour, how this happens and the way in which your body responds.

Your 'due date' can cause some anxiety and pressure, and it is important to keep in mind that everyone will have an individual gestational period, with 37–42 weeks being considered a normal window to give birth in. Only around 5 per cent of babies are born on their estimated due date so we need to ditch the due date pressure.

It is thought that labour is triggered by your baby releasing a small amount of a substance (surfactant protein) from their lungs that signals to your body that they are ready to be born. This then causes labour hormones to surge and labour to start.

There are a lot of myths about how to encourage labour to start and many are best avoided. However, there are a few natural physical preparation options that do have some evidence backing them up.

Raspberry leaf tea

The red raspberry leaves found in raspberry leaf tea have been shown to have a positive effect on labour. It is thought to work by strengthening the muscles of your uterus and the tea has been shown to shorten the length of labour (this is a big win if you ask me!) and reduce the likelihood of needing to have your waters broken, also making the chance of needing intervention for birth like forceps and caesarean less likely (we will discuss types of birth in Part 2). You can begin sipping two cups of red raspberry leaf tea daily from 32 weeks of pregnancy to help the compounds build up in your body to strengthen your uterus.

If you are planning a caesarean section birth, are pregnant with more than one baby, have a breech (bottom-first) baby, have high blood pressure or are taking metformin or antidepressants, it is advised to avoid raspberry leaf tea.

Eating dates

Dates are thought to have an oxytocin-like effect on your body, which can make your uterus more responsive to oxytocin in labour (who knew these shrivelled fruits could be so clever). Eating six dates daily from 36 weeks of pregnancy (skip this if you have gestational diabetes) may increase cervical ripening and reduce the need for induction. Women who ate dates were 74 per cent more dilated than those who didn't at the start of labour. Date eaters were also 21 per cent more likely to spontaneously go into labour and had a 77 per cent shorter first stage of labour. One small study also found dates reduced post-birth bleeding too. You're not going to get constipated getting all that fibre in either! A week into my date-eating mission in pregnancy I needed to liven them up a bit so I stuffed them with peanut butter and had them as a pudding.

Colostrum harvesting

Colostrum harvesting simply means using your hands to squeeze out and collect drops of colostrum (the very first milk that your body starts making in the second trimester). Colostrum harvesting can be done from 36 weeks using small 1-ml oral syringes and any collected can be frozen. Scan the QR code on page 6 for a guide on how to harvest colostrum. Doing this can be helpful if you are able to collect some colostrum and freeze it for when your baby arrives, but it may also increase your natural oxytocin levels, which helps your cervix prepare for labour.

Good sex

Sex has a duo of potential benefits when it comes to preparing for labour. Firstly, an orgasm triggers oxytocin, which you will remember from Chapter 2 is essential for labour. But it is also thought that semen may contain natural prostaglandins which help soften the cervix. Sex should be avoided if you've been advised to do so by your healthcare practitioner or once your waters have broken.

Clary sage essential oil

Clary sage is thought to stimulate your uterus to encourage contractions, so it is not recommended until your due date. You can mix a few drops with a carrier oil (or into a spoonful of full-fat milk to emulsify) for a bath or a few drops diluted into a room diffuser. You should avoid this if you have any pregnancy complications, and don't add it to a bath once your waters have broken.

PAUSE FOR THOUGHT

What three things can you do that are achievable for you to boost your physical birth preparation? For example, can you swap your office chair for a pregnancy ball to sit on? Can you download the NHS Squeezy App (see page 311) and commit to two rounds of pelvic floor exercises per day? Or can you add in an extra serving of an iron-rich food into your diet?

As you consider your physical preparation, also remember to keep your breathwork practice going strong. Trust in the hormonal dance between your body and your baby to trigger the start of labour and know that your baby will come when they are ready.

You have now got all of the essential physical and psychological tools and techniques you need to shape your birth powerfully and positively. Next we are going to talk about the locations available to you for birth and how your birthing space is going to serve you on this journey.

REMEMBER:

- Adopt upright and forward positions, and avoid slouching back in your sofa and chair for long periods to encourage your baby into an optimal position.
- Pelvic floor exercises are crucial during pregnancy and beyond. If you are not sure you are correctly performing them or have symptoms of pelvic dysfunction, ask your GP or midwife to refer you to a pelvic health specialist.
- Your baby will signal to your body when they are ready to be born, so do not allow your due date to cause anxiety or pressure.

5

CREATING YOUR POSITIVE BIRTH ENVIRONMENT

Your birth environment can often be considered an optional add-on, a 'nice if you can' or maybe even something that expectant parents don't plan for at all. In this chapter, I am going to challenge this perception and honour the importance of the environment during your labour. Your birth environment has been shown to have a positive impact on physiological birth and to improve your overall birth experience, helping you to achieve that positive and empowered start to parenthood.

If a feeling of control is an important consideration for you during birth, then environment is a great focus because, regardless of the building or location in which you birth, you can create a bubble within this that you can control and keep stable.

YOUR CHOICE OF BIRTH LOCATION

When it comes to deciding where to give birth, you'll usually have three options:

1. At home (home birth).
2. Midwife-led unit (located in the community) or a co-located midwife-led unit (inside the hospital).
3. Consultant-led unit (inside the hospital) – sometimes also called the labour ward or delivery suite.

Your obstetrician or midwife may advise on the recommended place for you to birth based on your medical and pregnancy history, and this may change throughout your pregnancy and even during labour. But ultimately it is your choice where you birth.

When choosing your birthing location, what is important is that you have a consultation with your team ahead of time to ensure you have all the best information available so you can be fully informed of the risks and benefits to each option and make a balanced, informed choice for you and your baby. If you wish to birth in a location that is not the recommended place for you based on guidelines and policies, you can make an informed decision to do this and this should be communicated to the team that will be caring for you so they understand and can support your wishes. It is your body and your baby; you are the boss.

The Birth Place Study in 2012 looked at different places in which women gave birth and which was safest for mums and babies. The findings showed that, for first-time mums with uncomplicated pregnancies, a midwife-led unit was safest, and for women who had had a baby before, home birth was associated with fewer medical interventions and no difference in health outcomes. Home birth for first-time mums also showed fewer medical interventions, but did also show poorer perinatal outcomes.

Midwife-led unit

If your pregnancy has been uncomplicated and you have only been seeing your midwife in a midwife-led care model, then the recommendation is to birth at home or in a midwife-led unit.

You can access many different forms of pain relief and use a birthing pool on a midwife-led unit, which we will discuss further in Part 2. The only option not available here would be an epidural. An epidural is a form of anaesthetic that interrupts pain signals between your spine and your brain. It can be a very effective form of pain relief for labour, but it does require some additional monitoring for you and your baby, which is why it is only available in a labour ward setting. We will discuss all the pain relief and comfort options available to you in Chapter 13.

Home birth

Home birth is typically only recommended when your pregnancy has been uncomplicated. When birthing at home, your midwives come to your home rather than you attending a birthing unit. You still have the same pain relief options and heart-rate monitoring available as you would in a midwife-led unit, but you would need to look at birthing pool hire if you wish to use one and the pain relief known as pethidine (see page 196) would need some prior planning.

Because you do need to plan for a home birth, your midwife will usually visit you at home in pregnancy to complete a home birth assessment. This allows them to understand your wishes and also note practicalities such as access to your home and parking, for example, so your team are well-prepared when the time comes.

Consultant-led unit (labour ward)

If you have been under the care of a consultant obstetrician and there have been some complications in your pregnancy, such as high blood pressure, pre-eclampsia, obstetric cholestasis, gestational diabetes or concerns over your baby's growth, to name a few, then you will likely be recommended to birth on a consultant-led unit. On a consultant-led unit you and your baby have quicker access to specialist doctors, medication and additional means of monitoring your baby. As mentioned above, an epidural (see page 197) is also only available on a consultant-led unit. Many consultant-led units have access to a birthing pool now and, if this is something that is important to you, you can ask your community midwife whether this is the case.

MONITORING YOU AND YOUR BABY IN LABOUR

The way in which your baby can be monitored during labour differs in different settings, and this is often the primary reason for your team recommending a given birth setting to you.

Your body and baby undergo a huge amount of work together during labour and birth. For many, each stage will progress smoothly without hiccup, but some women and babies experience a few twists and turns, and additional monitoring may be advised to ensure you and your baby are coping well with the process of labour.

During your pregnancy you may have heard your baby's heartbeat in a couple of ways – via a Sonicaid, is a small handheld machine that your midwife places on your stomach intermittently to listen to your baby's heart rate, or via a Cardiotocograph (CTG) monitor that prints out a trace of your baby's heartbeat. During established labour these same techniques are used to monitor your baby's well-being.

A Sonicaid is used in home birth or midwife-led settings. The use of this method is referred to as 'intermittent auscultation'. This means the handheld device is placed on to your abdomen for 1 minute and your midwife will count your baby's heartbeat – this happens every 15 minutes in the first stage of labour and every 5 minutes in the second stage. The monitoring of your baby's heartbeat is more frequent in the second stage because this is when babies are more likely to become distressed.

The CTG monitoring on a consultant-led unit allows your baby's heartbeat to be continuously monitoring by two round probes attached to your stomach with elastic belts. You can continue to be upright and mobile, but these monitors remain on for the duration of your labour until your baby is born. There is a big myth that, if you are continuously monitored during labour, you must be on a bed – you do not need to be left on a bed for continuous monitoring to happen. I repeat: you do not need to lie on a bed! Sometimes there are difficulties continuously monitoring your baby through your tummy. In these situations, a foetal scalp electrode (FSE) may be offered, which is a small clip that can attach to your baby's head and on to the CTG machine.

CTG monitoring has been criticised as, when it was introduced back in the sixties, the aim was that it would reduce the amount of babies who suffer complications from birth, but its use hasn't yet improved stillbirth rates or longer-term outcomes for babies, such as cerebral palsy. CTG use has reduced the number of babies experiencing seizures, but has also been linked to rising numbers of assisted vaginal or caesarean section births. When deciding on the recommended way to monitor your baby, your midwife or obstetrician will be able to explain to you what tools they have available, the evidence to support their recommendation and how that fits into your unique circumstance for your pregnancy and birth.

Your well-being throughout labour is vital too – if you are not well this can have a direct impact on how your little one manages labour. You will have monitoring for your blood pressure, signs of infection, signs of dehydration and rate of contractions, to name a few. Your midwife will conduct all this as discreetly as possible to help you remain in your calm birth bubble without interference.

WHY YOU MAY BE RECOMMENDED INTERMITTENT OR CONTINUOUS MONITORING IN LABOUR

A well-grown, full-term baby without complications going into labour is a baby with a full tank of oxygen, like a diver. They can tolerate a good amount of time in labour before their oxygen stores are depleted and they start to show any signs of being unwell. We monitor them closely with the handheld Sonicaid, but we do not need to monitor them continuously. If there have been some concerns or complications in your pregnancy, we can think of your baby as starting their labour journey with less oxygen or reserves in their tank. We are aware they could become unwell sooner and need to monitor them closely, so continuous CTG monitoring is advised during labour.

Remember, most babies manage labour without any problems, but for those who need a little extra monitoring or intervention, it is good to know that these options are available.

Vaginal examinations

Another form of monitoring is vaginal examinations (VEs). These may be offered to you for a variety of reasons, such as helping to determine the stage of labour you are in, how your labour is progressing by feeling for changes such as the softening, shortening and opening of your cervix, and the position and station (how low in your pelvis) your baby is in. During labour, a VE is typically offered every 4 hours, and the anticipated progress is 2cm dilation in this time. This is very much a guide and, although VEs have their place in labour, they really are not the whole picture, so I would encourage you not to get too caught up in how many centimetres dilated your cervix is as this can bring unnecessary anxiety. We must also remember that a VE gives us a snapshot at that moment and is a subjective measure – it is not uncommon for a woman to be 3cm dilated and, within 10 minutes, be having a baby. Findings on a VE are not the be-all and end-all, but they can be a useful piece to the puzzle.

A VE involves your midwife or obstetrician inserting two fingers into your vagina to your cervix. Some women will describe a VE as merely a little uncomfortable whereas others experience them as being more painful. Analgesia (pain relief) such as Entonox (gas and air – see page 195) can be provided for a VE should you wish. For women who have had previous difficult or traumatic sexual experiences or sexual assault, the idea of a VE can be quite distressing. If this is you, please speak with your team to seek their support and discuss your options. Utilising your breathing, visualisations and relaxed jaw (see Chapter 3) are all helpful ways for staying relaxed and calm during a VE in labour should you have one. Once your waters have broken, your midwife will be extra cautious on performing VEs as they have been linked to an increased risk of infection (see page 118).

VEs should be performed in a gentle, careful way and can be stopped at any point if you say so. VEs should only be performed with your informed consent, without any coercion, and this means you understanding the rationale behind the examination and being comfortable with it being performed. It is your body and nothing can be done to you without consent or continued if you say stop – to do so would be abuse.

Your vagina, your rules.

As a guide, I like to ask, 'Will the findings of this VE change anything we are doing?' If not, what's the point? If yes, it may be a useful option if you also agree. Some women find it reassuring to know what changes their cervix and baby have made, whereas other women find their oxytocin and adrenaline balance is disrupted by VEs – it is personal to you.

Fascinatingly, during labour, women develop a purple line or darkening of their skin colour from the base of their bottom that extends up the lower back as labour progresses. This is easier to notice on different skin colours, but is a non-invasive tool your midwife can use to check progress.

If you are ever unsure why a particular form of monitoring or intervention is being recommended to you, it is important to ask your team – they are on your side and will be more than happy to explain in more detail for you. This ensures informed consent, empowerment and control to you, but it is also really incredible what your body and baby are capable of, and it helps you to understand the processes happening too, which are just amazing.

'I am proud of myself, however my birth goes.'

YOUR BIRTH ENVIRONMENT

It is useful to consider the building where you birth – whether that is at home, in a birthing centre or on a labour ward – as merely being four walls around you. It is creating your ideal birth environment within these walls that will have the largest impact on your positive birth experience. This is your birth space bubble, and you can pick up this bubble and move it wherever you may need to.

It is important to feel relaxed and calm in your birthing environment. Feeling relaxed promotes oxytocin production, the hormone responsible for uterine contractions, and suppresses adrenaline, the hormone responsible for directing blood away from your uterus and inhibiting contractions. This is where the fight-or-flight response that we discussed in Chapter 1 becomes prominent (see page 13). If we feel unsafe, scared or fearful, our contractions and therefore the ability for our labour to progress normally are reduced as our adrenaline levels soar and our oxytocin levels are lowered.

The whole aim of your birth environment is to create a space and atmosphere that feels comfortable to you – this will of course feel different to each one of us as we are all so wonderfully unique. My first tip is to think about who you want at your birth and make sure it is someone you trust, who will support you and help you stay calm and relaxed.

The role of a birth partner may be taken on by a partner, family member or friend, someone whom you feel calm and relaxed around and who you trust. Of course, your midwife during labour and birth will also be providing you with support, but if they need to arrange medication or perform important checks and monitoring, this can interfere with their ability to provide the support basics, so having someone else there to help is of great benefit. Some women may choose to hire someone called a doula to support them during labour. A doula is a non-medically trained support person who can provide practical and emotional support during labour, but they cannot provide medical advice or care – see them as more of a birth coach.

Birthing partners are so important and continuous support in labour has been shown to reduce the need for pain relief or labour intervention.

All power to the birth partner – if they aren't already reading this book, then earmark this page for them! I have also dedicated a whole chapter to birth partners (Chapter 15) as they are so crucial.

Think about restricting the use of your mobile phone and maybe decide who, if anyone, you tell that you are in labour. Of course, your friends and family are excited for you and want to know what is happening, but constant messaging can interfere with your environment, so it can be a good idea to silence your phone and reassure them that you won't forget to tell them about the birth of your baby when it happens.

I recommend thinking about breaking down your birth environment into your five senses. I am shouting from the rooftops here that all these elements that create your all-important environment are transferrable into *any* setting. Communicating what you wish your environment to look, feel and sound like to your birth partner(s) means they can take care of this for you, and you can keep your brain in its primal state where it can best navigate the hormonal dance of birth.

The feeling in theatre was joyful. Everyone was smiling, chatting and laughing together – everyone was just so nice! Within what felt like minutes we were asked 'Are you ready?' and the drapes were lowered just in time for us to see our son enter the world. My bump was in the way so we saw nothing else but his face appearing, and shortly after we found out we had a son. We watched him take his first breath and, in that moment, he took ours away.

I can't even begin to describe the beauty of that moment and I feel so incredibly grateful we got to experience it. As he was placed on my chest it was like we were the only three people in the world.

Amelia

Consider each of your senses and what will make you feel safe, calm, in control and empowered, regardless of any twists and turns your labour may take:

Sight

Pack some battery candles or a little mood light (or both!) and dim the lights in your room. There may be some circumstances where it is medically necessary to have brighter lights on, but it is not routinely necessary for birth and, even in a theatre, the lighting can be dimmed, so speak with your team about your preferences around this. Having an eye mask to hand that you can pop on when lighting cannot be dimmed or simply closing your eyes is a handy tip for keeping this sense consistent.

Smell

Aromatherapy or room sprays that make you feel relaxed help create a calming space. Lots of hospitals offer an aromatherapy service now too, so have a chat about the options if you are interested in this. Essential oils can be used to relax you or even to help stimulate contractions. Oils such as lavender and frankincense are used for reducing tension and creating calm and relaxation. Peppermint oil can be used to help with nausea symptoms during labour. Sweet orange and jasmine are uplifting, mood-enhancing scents and clary sage is used to encourage more powerful contractions. Different oils and blends of oils may better suit different situations, so have a chat with your team about this if essential oils are of interest to you. Some oils are contraindicated in some circumstances, so always use aromatherapy under the support of someone trained in the practice. If you are using an eye mask then adding some lavender spray can be lovely and relaxing.

Sound

Create a playlist. Some women like to have a few options to choose from depending on the mood they wish to create. A calm, relaxing playlist for the first stage of labour and a motivating, empowering playlist for the second stage works well for some, whereas other woman like to keep it all chilled. I have supported women listening to whale sounds and others listening to hard rock tunes – you do what works for you, but don't rely on someone else to create this for you unless they know you very well because it is so personal. You can play your music directly from your phone or bring along a small speaker or headphones.

Taste

Pack up all the snacks! Food is a very emotive thing so have foods that you enjoy and that will give you energy for labour and birth. Little nibbles work best, so think energy sweets, cereal bars or crackers, not three-course meals. You could make some snacks of your own to take in – dates stuffed with nut butter, mini sandwich bites or banana loaf all work well. When planning your labour snacks, think easy to store and easy to eat. Having a mixture of sweet and savoury is a wise move, as often women pack lots of sweet options and then get a bit sick of sweet flavours a few hours in. Some women find it a challenge to eat in labour and, as long as you're hydrated, your body will be OK without food for a period of time, but the earlier stages, when you are more likely to feel you can eat, are a great opportunity to fuel up. Remember, too, birthing your baby is an event to be celebrated, so have a special something for that post-birth cuddle to indulge in. Somehow I managed to put away a plate of chilli con carne, a sticky toffee pudding, half a pack of chocolate Hobnobs and an Indian takeaway after giving birth – turns out it is hungry work.

Touch

If you are birthing in a midwife- or consultant-led unit, bring a comfy pillow so you aren't relying on pancake-flat hospital ones. I recommend packing a flannel too for your birth partner to use to cool you down during labour – a cool flannel over your forehead or the back of your neck can feel wonderful. You can even use your flannel with essential oils on to inhale all the relaxing, soothing scents. A handheld fan or water spray bottle can also work well.

Wear something comfortable, that you can move freely in and that feels nice against your skin. An oversized T-shirt or stretchy loungewear are good options and, of course, something to wear in water if you plan to use the pool. Some women prefer to be naked during labour, especially if it is a warm day, and that is fine too, but having options is a sensible move. When I look back at photos, I was one for the fashion police in labour: leggings with a giant bright blue T-shirt finished off with a knitted cardigan/dressing gown. It was an interesting look, but I was comfy and ended up in a sports bra in the pool eventually.

Also think about packing some soft, comfy socks or a massage tool that your birth partner can use to help keep you comfortable. Some women like light touch and find massage helpful, whereas others like to be in water. Everyone feels different about touch and while some find it comforting in labour, others do not want to be touched at all – you probably know where you stand on this and you can talk to your birthing partner about your touch preferences.

MY TOP TEN LABOUR COMFORTS

Simple comforts in labour are easily underestimated, but the most basic things can be game changing. Here are my top ten simple labour comforts to add to your hospital bag:

1. Lip balm: hospital air-conditioning systems and Entonox (gas and air) can really dry out lips.
2. Cooling water spray: labour is warm work.
3. Hairbands/clips: to keep your hair out of your face.
4. Extra-long phone-charging cable: so you can reach your mobile while it is charging.
5. A water bottle with a straw: easy-access hydration from lots of positions.
6. A dirty laundry bag: makes for much easier unpacking.
7. A mood light or battery candles: because hopefully I have sold you on how important environment is.
8. A wooden comb: for acupressure pain relief (I will talk you through this in Chapter 13).
9. Affirmations: these could be written on Post-it notes to pop around the room or get crafty with pretty cards, but keep those positive, confidence-boosting words close by.
10. Your favourite toiletries: that post-birth wash is pure heaven and you deserve a mini pamper.

Chat with your birthing partner well before labour so they can help manage this all for you.

I really encourage you to use your senses to help shape your birth environment vision when you complete your birth preference plan (page 223) – your oxytocin levels will be eternally grateful.

The atmosphere you create in your birthing room is much more important and influential on your birth than the precise location. I encourage you to not get too caught up with the building you birth in, but to embrace the control over what your space looks and feels like instead.

In the next chapter, we are going to discuss how to make truly informed decisions around your birth.

REMEMBER:

- If you do not understand or feel entirely comfortable with a form of monitoring offered to you, have a conversation with your care provider so you can make informed decisions around this part of your care.
- Create a birthing bubble based on your senses that you can use in any birth space.
- Communicate your birth environment preferences to your birth partner and allow them to take the lead on facilitating it so you can focus on your priority of managing each contraction.

6

MAKING INFORMED DECISIONS TO BE YOUR BIRTH BOSS

Pregnancy, birth and parenthood present a series of decision-making hurdles, and navigating your options can feel overwhelming at times. In this chapter I will empower you with information and tools to help you to make informed decisions that you feel are best for you and your baby – in partnership with your care providers. I have included this early on in the book so you can utilise the tools as you move through the book and learn more about your different birth options, such as your choices around induction of labour, pain relief remedies and the different types of birth.

INFORMED CONSENT AND BIRTH RIGHTS

Informed consent is a process by which your healthcare practitioner must provide you with the risks, benefits and any alternatives to a procedure or intervention. It is an ethical and legal obligation to ensure you are well-informed, without bias or coercion to make a decision about your body. You can then choose to accept or decline the procedure or intervention through informed decision-making. If you accept, you are giving informed consent and the procedure or intervention can happen, and if you decline, you are declining to give consent and the procedure or intervention won't happen. You can always ask for more time to make a decision or for more information, and you can also change your mind about the choice you make. In law, a baby doesn't have any rights until it is born, so during pregnancy and birth, even if your medical team feel something should happen to protect your unborn baby and where you have mental capacity, they cannot act without your consent.

When giving birth you have birth rights – seven key human rights within the maternity system (also check out the Birthrights website on page 311 for more information). These are:

1. You have the right to be treated with dignity and respect at all times.
2. You always have the right to say no.
3. When you ask for care, maternity services must start from 'yes' and only say no if they have a good reason.
4. You have the right to have all your basic needs met.
5. You have the right to be supported and to be together as a family.
6. You have the right to complain.
7. You always have the right to receive care.

Your team, your midwife, your doctors and obstetrician are all there to support you and, like you, they want the best, safest and most positive outcome and experience for you and your baby. You are one big team and, as the expectant mum in the team, you are at the centre, and every suggestion and decision is made with you in mind. I encourage you to embrace the expertise on hand, express your wishes and be open to conversations unpicking potential interventions should they crop up.

I took opportunities to ask questions and discuss the various birth options, and the pros and cons to each. It meant I was able to have better and more informed discussions with the doctors and actually found that the medical professionals were really receptive to my questions as I understood what they were suggesting and could discuss what was best for me. I was so confident going into birth that I didn't write a birth plan. I had an ideal scenario in my mind, but I felt equipped with enough knowledge to make decisions on the go.

Sarah

WEIGHING UP YOUR OPTIONS

It's important to remember that you, your baby and your circumstances are all unique and individual. What may feel like the right decision for your friend may be different for you, so try to avoid comparing your choices and decisions to those of others around you and try to silence the sea of differing opinions you will inevitably see online. Instead, try to focus on ensuring decisions are made from an informed place. The two tools below will help you to weigh up your options and make the decision that is right for you and your baby.

The Scales tool

Imagine you have a set of old-fashioned weighing scales. With every decision you make, you are weighing up the risks against the benefits or the pros against the cons specific to you and your circumstances. The scales tip to one option or the other for you.

You will already be doing this automatically in your day-to-day life: 'Do we get a takeaway tonight?' 'Should I buy this dress or that dress?' 'Should we go on a family holiday?' Your brain is used to functioning in this way, but when it comes to pregnancy and birth choices, often there is more at stake, more information to gather and questions to ask. It is a new field for you, and having a structured approach is really helpful. The Scales tool gives you a quick, almost instinctive balance and encourages you to ask questions and gather more information. Know that your health-care provider, midwife or obstetrician will be happy to answer any questions you may have and/or signpost you to additional resources. Sometimes it can be challenging to remember all your queries in an appointment, so consider writing them down ahead of time so you can easily remember them. Recognise that this process can be a team effort that needs flexibility and understanding from all involved. And that, ultimately, you are the boss of your birth.

This tool may be enough to support your decision-making or you may need to dig a little deeper with the BRAIN tool below.

Use your BRAIN

This is a simple acronym to keep handy for any of life's small or larger decisions over the next weeks and months, and it is a solid, sure way to make informed decisions:

- Benefits: what are the benefits?
- Risks: what are any associated risks?
- Alternatives: what are the alternatives?
- Intuition: what is my intuition telling me?
- Nothing: what happens if I do nothing?

You can use this for anything from what to have for dinner to where to birth your baby. It is also a fantastic tool for birth partners to use when advocating for you during birth. See pages 164, 200 and 219 for examples of the BRAIN tool in action.

Unfortunately, especially through the medium of social media, medical intervention is often demonised, but it's important we do not see it as the enemy. The reality is that appropriate use of inter-vention saves lives and is the reason mortality in childbirth is as low as it is in today's world. Your midwife and obstetrician won't rec-ommend intervention without any reason. But what is crucial is that you understand this reason, explore it and are supported to make the right choice for you. This is where the use of the Scales and the BRAIN tools are helpful and will provide you with the prompts you need to reach your decision.

Remember, it's your body and your baby, the control and final decisions are always in your hands. Your team are on your side and will hold a safe space for you to ask questions, have open, honest and judgement-free discussions to ultimately empower you.

> *There were a couple of unexpected hurdles throughout my pregnancy, one of which was that, during my third trimester, Doppler readings showed reduced blood flow through my placenta and a slowing in my baby's growth. I was advised that I should be induced before 36 weeks. I was informed with expert knowledge to understand the induction process. This empowered me to ask questions and weigh up the risks using the BRAIN tool.*
>
> Jessica

Grab some paper and try this tool with something about your pregnancy or birth that you have been deliberating to see how it helps.

INTERPRETING STATISTICS

It is important to consider statistics and how these can be presented when making decisions. For example, you may see that a risk or chance of a certain outcome *doubles*. Doubling sounds large and scary and may influence your decision in one way or the other. However, it is important you feel able to examine this further and the way to do this is to ask for numerical values instead. For example, you may be told that a risk doubles, but the stats show this is from 0.2 to 0.4 per cent. Have a think about how 'double the risk' compares in this instance. Would your decision change?

Again, there is no right or wrong, but having real, numerical values means you can ensure you are making informed decisions. What will feel like a comfortable degree of risk for one woman, will feel too much for another. Decisions, as a result, will vary – pregnancy and birth are not black and white and there is no one-size-fits-all solution.

'I'm prepared to meet any turns and changes my body and baby take during this process.'

Adding the ability to make informed decisions to the birth preparation we have previously discussed allows you to have confidence that, even if your birth deviates from the smoothest path or some twists or turns crop up, you have the power to be adaptive and have a positive journey still.

The next step is packing your hospital bag so you have all the physical items ready to go too.

REMEMBER:

- You have the right to be made aware of all risks, benefits and alternatives available to you.
- It is OK to decline a recommendation; just ensure you have a comprehensive understanding of why it was recommended and are happy with the risk versus benefits balance.
- Remember to use your old-fashioned scales to weigh up the pros and cons for you and your BRAIN tool when making decisions.

7

PACKING YOUR HOSPITAL BAG MADE EASY

As you get towards your estimated due date, one of the things you will be pondering is when to pack your hospital bag and what to put in it. There is nothing as frustrating as forgetting that one much-needed item, and no one wants to be packing their bag while going into labour, so being organised is key.

In my experience, packing the bag is often a task that occupies more energy and time of expectant parents than it needs to and can be an overwhelming job, so I am going to make it stress-free by breaking things down, simplifying it and helping you to have a well-organised bag ensuring none of your essentials get left behind. I am also going to share with you my complete hospital bag check-list so you can confidently labour knowing you have everything you need to hand.

The first thing to consider is *when* to pack the bag. Remember, a baby is considered full-term from 37 weeks, but it is also common to still be pregnant beyond your estimated due date. This means that your little one could make an appearance any time between 37 and 42 weeks, and this is considered a very normal window in which your baby can be born. Of course, there are some babies who decide to make a slightly earlier entrance into the world, so it is a good idea to have your bag packed from around 35–36 weeks. However, any earlier than this and you may be like me ahead of packing for a holiday, when you forget what you have actually packed because you did it so long ago.

Now, this is a sneaky midwife insider tip: it isn't usually you (mum) who is getting things out of the bag, especially during labour. It is more likely to be your birth partner or midwife, so you may want to pack in a way that protects your perfectly packed bag from ending up strewn all over your birth room floor in a desperate rush to locate a specific item in your time of need.

It also worth bearing in mind who you are packing for: mum, birth partner(s) and baby . . . or babies! This leads to my first bit of advice: encourage your birth partner to get involved in the packing so they know where to find things. Then, for ultimate ease of packing and unpacking, think about having a separate bag or separate section of the bag for your baby's things so you aren't hunting through nappies for your lip balm or babygrows for your post-birth underwear.

There is no right or wrong type of bag to use. I would try to utilise a weekend bag or small suitcase you have already, so it doesn't become an added expense. Then, have a separate birth partner bag so they can easily access all their essentials and keep themselves fed without disturbing you or rummaging through your bag. A rucksack is a good idea for this as it can be carried on their back when you leave the hospital and their arms are full of you, baby and your other bags.

My next bit of advice for making things easy is labelling. Make life super simple and put your items into transparent bags that you can stick a label on – for example, muslins, baby's first outfit, going home outfit, post-birth underwear and PJs – before placing them in your hospital bag. Labelling like this is especially useful if you are taking in clothing for your baby in a couple of different sizes as it means there is no fiddling through clothes labels to check which size is which. You can have one smaller bag of newborn size and one of 0–3 months, for example. That being said, most newborn sleepsuits will fit babies up to around 9–10 pounds.

It's also a good idea to pack a separate bag for clothing that gets dirty and used in hospital, so you don't have baby poo stains mixing with your clean items. This way, when you get home, weary-eyed and in need of your own bed, you can take the dirty bag out and know the rest of the unpacking can wait (or, even better, be done by someone else).

And before we get into what items to pack, remember you are unlikely to be in hospital for very long. A typical postpartum stay varies from six hours to just a few days, so you don't need to pack for a two-week holiday. Your unpacking self will thank you for keeping it to just the minimum essentials.

Once all packed, leave your bag by the front door so you don't forget it on the day or night. If you are planning to birth at home, I recommend having a transfer bag ready so that, should you need to go into hospital for some reason, you don't use energy finding things to pack up in a hurry.

I've included a checklist of essentials for you below (you're welcome – in return, please complete a round of birth breaths and pelvic floor exercises!).

HOSPITAL BAG ESSENTIALS

Baby

- A few, perhaps three, sleepsuits
- Around three bodysuits or vests depending on the temperature and time of year
- A hat

- A cardigan if it is cooler outside
- A snowsuit for going home if it is cold outside
- A few muslins
- A blanket
- Plenty of nappies: a pack of 20 is a good idea
- Cotton wool or fragrance-free wipes if this is your preference
- Car seat

Mum: in labour

- Maternity notes
- Your birth plan: we will cover more on this on page 223
- Your playlist/music/speakers
- TENS machine (see page 193) if planning to use
- Clothing to birth in that is comfortable and allows you to move freely
- A comfortable pillow
- Some entertainment: a pack of cards, music, phone charger, books, etc.
- Lots and lots of snacks (see page 90)
- A sports water bottle
- A flannel
- A wash bag and toiletries

See also page 92 for my top ten labour comforts, which you may also choose to include.

Mum: after birth

- Large cotton knickers: around five pairs
- A pack of maternity pads

- A comfortable bra. If planning to breastfeed, choose a nursing-style bra
- Slippers or flip-flops
- Dressing gown
- Comfortable nightwear
- Comfortable day outfit to wear home
- An extra-long phone-charging cable
- Some cash or a card for paying for parking or a trip to the shop if you fancy it

Birth partner

- Lots of snacks too: no one wants a hangry birth partner. They should also make sure they keep themselves hydrated and fuelled.
- Again, some cash or card to pay for parking and café trips
- A change of clothes
- A simple wash bag to keep them feeling fresh
- Some entertainment, such as a book or podcast

Breaking it down into who and when you're packing for really does make the unpacking a lot easier and simpler. This means that you can spend more time snuggling your little one and less time rummaging through bags.

NEW BABY CHECKLIST

While we are on the subject of lists to make your life easier, you may have been pondering what you actually need to get ready for your baby, so I have laid this all out here for you too . . .

Equipment

- Car seat
- Pram
- Crib/Moses basket
  Safe sleeping advice is that your baby sleeps in the same room as you for the first six months of life (both day and night), so consider how this will work in your home.
- Mattress and waterproof protector
- Cot sheets x 2–4
- Baby carrier/sling
- Baby towels x 2
- Blankets x 2–4
- Muslins x 8–10
- Play mat and soft toy
  Newborns don't need lots of toys but remember they can only see high-contrast colours to start with, so bear this in mind when choosing books and toys.
- Baby bath
- Thermometers
  One to check your baby's temperature, one to check room temperature and one for the bath.
- Changing mat
  One for home, but a travel one for your changing bag is also handy.
- Changing bag

Baby clothing

*A note on baby clothing: sizes vary between brands but, generally, newborn size fits a baby up to about 10 pounds. They tend to outgrow this size very quickly and larger babies may fit into 0–3 months at birth.

- Vests x 8–10
  These may be sleeveless, short-sleeved or long-sleeved depending on the season in which your baby is born.
- Babygrows (also called sleep suits) x 8–10
- Outfits x 2
  You may choose to leave this out and stick with baby-grows. It's your personal choice. If using socks, check out 'sock ons' to help them stay on.
- Hats x 2
- Mittens x 2
  Specifically warm mittens if baby is born in the winter. Scratch mitts can be useful but many babygrows have these built in.
- Snowsuit
  Also called a pramsuit – not applicable to babies born in summer.
- Cardigans x 2

For Mum

- Hospital nightie/PJs
- Nursing bras/tops if breastfeeding
- Big cotton knickers for post-birth
- Maternity pads

Nappies/feeding

- Nappies and nappy bags

- Cotton wool/wipes
- Nappy cream
  Sudocrem and Metanium are great for treating nappy rash.

Depending on your feeding choice . . .
- Breast pads
- Nursing pillow
- Nipple cream (a lanolin-based cream such as Lansinoh)
- Breast pump and milk storage bags
- Bottles and teats
- Steriliser
- Infant formula

Please remember that the main thing your new baby needs is you – your love and attention as they navigate the world outside of your body. The materialistic things do not matter even half as much as you may think at the moment, so don't feel overwhelmed with lists of things to buy and, if you have forgotten something, you can always get it when your little one is here.

REMEMBER:

- You are packing your bag for you, your birth partner(s) and baby(s) – at least three people.
- Keep your birth environment bits within easy reach for your birth partner so when you arrive in your birth space they can create the environment you planned in Chapter 5.
- Include your favourite snacks and toiletries for a post-birth treat. Your baby's birth needs celebrating and you will benefit from simple luxuries.

PART 1
REFLECTION

Congratulations, you have completed Part 1. Hopefully you should be feeling empowered by your body and its capabilities on this journey. You truly are incredible! You now have tools and techniques to practise and reflect on as we continue into Part 2.

QUIZ

Here is your end of Part 1 quiz. This is a simple activity to help you consolidate all the information we have talked about so far and I really encourage you to give it a go to get the best from your birth preparation.

1. What is the breath for the first stage of labour?
2. What is the breath for the second stage of labour?
3. How long does a contraction last?
4. What hormone is predominantly working for your uterus to contract in labour?
5. From how many weeks can you start drinking raspberry leaf tea?
6. What is the minimum number of minutes of moderate-intensity exercise recommended per week in pregnancy?

---

7. From what gestation is colostrum harvesting recommended?

8. What are your two decision-making tools?

The quiz answers are on page 309 so you can check your new knowledge.

Jot down any key take-homes from Part 1 in the space below:

_____

_____

_____

_____

_____

_____

_____

_____

_____

_____

_____

_____

_____

PART 2
It's Time to Birth

We have discussed powerful psychological and physical birth preparation tools in Part 1 and it's now time to piece all of this information together and apply it to your actual birth. You'll come to recognise how birth can happen in many forms and each is as momentous and beautiful as the other. There is no one right way to birth your baby, but, when you do, these next chapters will help you feel that it is an empowering experience.

In this part, we'll explore the process of labour and birth, and all of the options and choices available to you on the journey. I encourage you to keep bringing your mind back to this important message as you read through the chapters that follow: We cannot control all the variables and there may well be elements of your birth that are not within your control. But there are aspects that you *can* influence and these will be the things that ensure, despite any potential twists or turns, that you feel like a superwoman when you bring your baby into the world.

Birth takes a woman's deepest fears about herself and shows her that she is stronger than all of them.

8

YOUR JOURNEY THROUGH LABOUR

Your journey through labour can be divided into five stages: the latent phase, the first stage, the transition stage, the second stage and the third stage. How you move through each is individual to you and your baby. Understanding these different parts of labour, when your waters may break and what is happening to your body can be super-reassuring, supports your mind to have confidence in your body and helps you know what practical things you can do to help your body and baby in each stage. So here is exactly what you need to know about your journey through labour and to welcoming your baby into your arms.

There are around 270 babies worldwide sharing the exact same minute of birth as your baby. You are going through this experience with hundreds of other women at the same time – you are not alone.

WHAT TO EXPECT WHEN YOUR WATERS BREAK

Your baby develops and grows inside a bag of water called the amniotic sac, which is filled with amniotic fluid, aka your 'waters'.

Initially, the amniotic fluid is water made from you, but by around halfway through your pregnancy it is made up of your growing baby's urine, and your baby swallows and excretes fluid into it. The level of amniotic fluid is highest at around 36 weeks, at approximately 800ml, then it reduces a little at 40 weeks to about 600ml (think of a standard cola bottle that is 500ml when trying to picture just how much fluid is in your uterus . . . impressive!). The level of amniotic fluid is one of the things checked on your ultrasound scans; too little is termed oligohydramnios and too much is called polyhydramnios. If either of these conditions is detected, you will be offered additional care and monitoring.

Amniotic fluid plays an important role for your growing baby during pregnancy:

- It acts like a shock absorber to protect your baby, like a protective cushioning.
- It provides your baby with insulation to keep them warm and to maintain a constant, regular temperature inside your uterus.
- It contains antibodies which help protect your baby against infections.
- By swallowing the amniotic fluid and using it to practise breathing, your baby uses the muscles within their lungs and digestive system, which helps them to develop.
- The liquid nature of amniotic fluid inside your uterus allows your baby to move freely. This movement supports the development of their muscles and bones.
- Adequate levels of fluid ensure that smaller body parts such as your baby's fingers and toes have lubrication to grow individually and not together, which causes webbing.

- It allows the umbilical cord to function optimally, as the fluid prevents the umbilical cord from being compressed which would reduce the flow of oxygen and nutrients through the placenta to your baby.

When the amniotic sac breaks or tears, this fluid leaks out via your cervix and vagina. This is not painful, but you may feel a 'pop' and gush of fluid, or you may just feel a slow trickle and leaking. Sometimes it is quite tricky to know for sure if your waters have broken and your midwife may recommend performing a speculum examination to work out if they have gone or not. The fluid will continue to trickle out once the sac has broken as amniotic fluid is continually made so that your baby always has fluid around them.

The amniotic sac may tear behind your baby – 'hindwaters' – or in front of your baby – 'forewaters'. Hindwaters tend to be associated with more of a trickle and forewaters with more of a pop and a gush. This is predominantly because your baby acts as a bit of a plug when your hindwaters break so less fluid can drain out. Scan the QR code on page 6 to understand this in a more visual way.

Your waters may break before or during labour, and some babies are even born in their sac of waters – known an 'en caul'. When your waters do break, it typically does not look like the movies where the waters go, flood everywhere and then there is a huge rush because the baby is coming. There is no need to rush or panic when your waters break – keep in that calm, controlled zone utilising all the techniques we talked through in Part 1: think breathing, visualisations, trust in your body and baby and use of affirmations.

I was sceptical as to how helpful breathing really could be in labour as it didn't especially resonate with me antenatally. I'd practised both up and down breathing, but couldn't really 'get into it'. As my contractions

> *intensified, I was surprised to find that up breathing helped to centre me as the contractions built and passed. I'm convinced that this helped me 'relax' and ultimately contributed to my labour progressing as quickly as it did.*
>
> Ali

Your waters should be clear or lightly straw-coloured, and they should not be green, brown or bright red and shouldn't have an offensive smell. It is a good idea to put a maternity pad in your underwear so you can monitor the fluid coming out, see the colour clearly and show your midwife. When amniotic fluid is red, it can indicate bleeding, which should prompt further monitoring of you and your baby. When it is green or brown, it indicates that baby has passed meconium (the name of their first poo) in the uterus.

Meconium isn't like poo as we know it – it is actually around 75 per cent water with amniotic fluid, mucous, skin cells, bile, hair and gut cells mixed in, and is a dark green, blacky colour and is sticky like Marmite (love it or hate it!). Meconium-stained fluid is pretty common and is seen in around 15–20 per cent of term babies and 30–40 per cent of babies born after their due date. Typically, the concern is less when a baby is term or post-term as their digestive system is mature and begins to move meconium. This maturity is not quite established in preterm babies, so the presence of meconium may be more concerning.

Meconium-stained fluid may present for different reasons and some of the theories include:

- The compression of a baby's head and umbilical cord during normal, physiological labour causes movement in their digestive tract, releasing meconium, so as a baby is born, a trail of meconium follows.

- Babies in a breech (bum-first) position may pass meconium that exits like toothpaste out of its tube due to the pressure as they move through the birth canal.
- In some cases, where mums have a pregnancy liver condition causing abnormal bile acids (intrahepatic cholestasis of pregnancy), more fluid travels through the baby's bowel and this may lead to meconium being passed.

Your team will ask to keep a closer eye on your baby if there is meconium in your waters to make sure it is not a sign that your baby is unwell inside. If there is low oxygen, babies' guts can be stimulated and their bottoms relaxed, which releases their poo into the waters. There are thought to be two types of meconium: thin, where it is just a very light tinge in your waters, or thick where it is much darker green or brown in colour. Generally, there is much less worry about thin meconium than thick meconium. This is because thicker meconium is more likely to be breathed in by a baby, although it is rare that this happens (only 2–3 per cent of the 15–20 per cent of babies with meconium-stained waters). This can cause a complication called meconium aspiration syndrome (MAS) if inhaled by baby and can make babies very unwell. For this reason, some additional care and monitoring may be recommended for you to reduce this risk.

If you think that your waters may have broken, it is recommended to call your midwife or local maternity unit. Often you will be invited in for a well-being check of you and your baby and to confirm whether your waters have indeed broken. After this, if there are no concerns and you are full-term (over 37 weeks) you will often go back home to wait for your contractions to start.

Your waters can break before or during labour. For 1 in 20 women the waters break before their contractions begin and it is reassuring to know that, when this happens, for most women (around 60–80 per cent) labour will start on its own within the next

24 hours. After 24 hours the likelihood of labour starting on its own reduces, but by 48 hours about 90 per cent of women will go into labour.

When your waters do break, you will be recommended to keep an eye on yourself for any signs of feeling unwell or feverish and on the colour of your waters that will keep leaking out. The reason for this is that there is some concern around longer intervals between waters breaking and birth because of an increasing chance of developing an infection (from 0.5 to 1 per cent at 24 hours). Your waters were like a protective balloon around your baby preventing infection from getting into your uterus, but, when there is an opening in this balloon of waters, infection could travel up the vagina and sneak in. Your team will keep any VEs to an absolute minimum because there is a correlation between more VEs and an increasing chance of infection, although this is most significant with over five VEs.

If you are full-term in your pregnancy when your waters break but labour has not yet started, you will be given some options:

- to have an induction of labour (see Chapter 11), or
- to await labour to start on its own and monitor – this is some-times called 'expectant management'

If your pregnancy is preterm (before 37 weeks) and your waters break, your team will have a discussion with you and make recommendations based on how many weeks you are exactly and your medical and pregnancy history. Often the aim is to closely monitor mum and baby for infection and aim for expectant management until 37 weeks, but each situation is unique to mum and will be discussed with you on an individual basis.

Another time when the plan may differ for you is if your waters break and you carry Group B strep (GBS). GBS is a common bacteria carried by 20–40 per cent of women in the UK. Most women who carry GBS will have no symptoms and it is not harmful to you if you do carry it, but there is a small chance it could cause an infection in your baby. About 1 in 400 babies born to a mother who is known to carry develops GBS infection in the UK. Currently, in the UK GBS testing is not routine in pregnancy and often it is found coincidentally on a vaginal swab or urine test. GBS can be transient in nature, meaning you can have it one week and not the next, which is one of the reasons why testing is a challenge as it may mean treating mums and babies who don't actually carry GBS at the time of birth and not treating those who then do carry it at the time of birth. If you did have GBS confirmed in pregnancy it is recommended to have intravenous antibiotics throughout your labour to help protect baby. This may limit your birth place choices. You can opt to pay for private testing (see Further Resources, page 311, for more information on this). It is recognised that prolonged (over 24 hours) rupture of membranes increases the chance of a baby becoming unwell with GBS infection, so you would be advised to commence labour induction if your labour didn't start spontaneously when your waters break and you were known to carry GBS.

The information I've outlined above highlights how there are many variables through pregnancy and your, and your baby's, journey is unique. Having reliable, evidence-based information like this enables you to make informed decisions during your pregnancy and birth.

Knowing where recommendations come from and having all the options available to you is really important in maintaining control and ensuring your experience is an informed and empowered one.

Using your Scales and BRAIN decision-making tools from Chapter 6 (see page 98) will allow you to make sure that you remember you are a birth boss.

THE LATENT PHASE

The latent phase of labour is the very beginning stage. It is essentially your body practising and preparing for labour, and can last anywhere from hours to multiple days, often stopping and starting, causing contractions irregularly and on and off. It is a key part of labour and your body makes many important changes during this stage.

Your cervix starts off as a long, firm, closed and tubular structure, and, during the latent phase, it becomes softer, thinner, moves to sit further forwards and begins to gently open. This process is called the effacement or ripening of the cervix. It is your cervix making its preparations to open during the next stage of labour.

You may experience some period-type pains, Braxton Hicks (see page 42) and the start of contractions, but they will often be short-lasting and irregular. They may even stop all together for a period of time before starting again.

At this stage, you may notice a 'show' or mucous plug. This is a jelly-like mucous substance that acts as a plug in your cervix during pregnancy to protect your baby from infection. As your cervix starts to change, this plug is dislodged and may come out. You might notice it in your underwear or when you wipe yourself after going to the toilet. It is usually thick and clear, almost a snotty consistency, and may have some streaks of blood in it. It doesn't tell you when exactly you will go into labour, but it is a positive sign that your body is preparing and it's not far off. Some women may never notice their mucous plug come away, while others may notice it for a few days.

If there are no medical issues and you are 37 weeks or over, then it is usually recommended that you stay at home for the latent stage to give labour the best chance of progressing naturally. This is a great time to tap into the positive birth environment that you planned out in Chapter 5, to get your oxytocin flowing and assist your body and baby to progress in labour. The upwards breathing technique you started to practise in Chapter 3 comes out to play in the latent phase of labour, so be ready to whip it out of your back pocket.

To help you stay positive and comfortable during the latent phase of labour, I recommend using the acronym READ:

- **R**est: The latent phase can be tiring and uncomfortable. Often contractions come on more at night-time, making it tricky to sleep. So, rest when you need to and nap if you can. Eating and drinking are really important – stay hydrated and nourished, and snack regularly! Your uterus is a muscle, and every tightening is your muscle contracting. It is important to keep these muscles fuelled, just as you would fuel your body for any other endurance event.

- **E**ase discomfort: Try a hot water bottle and warm baths – gentle heat and water can be really useful for managing symptoms that are often like menstrual cramps. You can safely take paracetamol in pregnancy if you have no contrain-dications, which will give you some gentle respite.

- **A**ctive: Try going for a walk or bouncing on your birthing ball to encourage labour to progress. Staying active helps encourage your body to move into 'established' labour by aiding the pressure of your baby's head on to your cervix. Also think about adopting the upright, forwards and open positions to help your baby be in an optimal position for birth that we discussed in Chapter 4 (we will be taking a deep dive into great positions you can use for birth in Chapter 12).

- **D**istraction: A lot of this phase is all about distraction and occu-pying your mind while your body does amazing things, so try listening to music, catching up on some TV, reading books or playing games on your phone. Baking a cake is also a great distraction technique, if that's your thing, and also means you have a birthday cake ready for when your baby is born – a win-win!

It is important to keep an eye on your baby's movement pattern during this stage. Your baby's movement pattern should stay the same in late pregnancy and in labour itself, so if you feel there is a change in any way from your baby's normal pattern or you have any concerns, it is important to call your local maternity unit or midwife to be checked over.

THE FIRST STAGE

The first stage of labour is often labelled as the 'established' or 'active' phase of labour. It means that your body has committed to birthing your baby from this point onwards and is fully warmed up and ready.

In this stage, your cervix has dilated to around 4cm and your contractions are powerful and regular, coming around every 3 minutes and each lasting for 40–60 seconds.

The first stage lasts from a cervical dilation of 4cm until your cervix is 10cm or fully dilated – this means it is all behind your baby's head.

For women having their first baby, the first stage usually lasts for about 8 hours and is rarely longer than 18 hours. For women who have had a baby before, the first stage usually lasts for about 5 hours and is rarely longer than 12 hours.

If you feel you are experiencing regular contractions coming every 3 minutes and about 40–60 seconds apart, then you are in the established phase of labour. You will need to call your home birth midwife, birthing centre or consultant-led unit (depending on where you plan to give birth – see Chapter 5) so that you can receive one-to-one care and support all the way through to the birth of your baby. The upwards breath (page 47) continues to serve as your most helpful sidekick throughout the first stage of labour, so be mindful of keeping this at the forefront as your contractions continue.

THE TRANSITION STAGE

As you approach full dilation, where your cervix is 10cm dilated, there is a period called transition, marking the time you transition from the first to the second stage of labour. For some women, this stage goes unnoticed, but for others they experience a change in their contractions and in their behaviour.

You may experience some physical symptoms, such as nausea or vomiting, or some emotional symptoms, such as a feeling of being overwhelmed or unable to cope. This stage can feel as though you have been cruising along in your car and then suddenly have to do an emergency stop – your adrenaline levels rise, and you need to take a moment to readjust before continuing on to complete your journey.

Recognising when you have hit the transition stage and that it is a completely normal part of the process can be very reassuring. Your birth partner can be really helpful in talking you through this stage. It is temporary and doesn't last much longer than around ten minutes and it means that you really are very close to meeting your baby.

Again, your upwards breath continues to support you in transition, although some women find it harder to maintain. Having a birthing partner who also knows this breath and can prompt you, ground you and support you to reconnect with it during this stage is really helpful.

THE SECOND STAGE

The second stage of labour is the stage when your cervix is fully dilated and your body is ready to birth your baby. It is the most exciting stage as it means that the birth of your baby is really close.

In this stage of labour, your upwards breath switches to your downwards breath (flick back to Chapter 3 if you need a quick reminder of the difference) because the goal in this stage is for your baby to move downwards to be born.

Remember: your body knows how to do this; your mind just needs to trust it!

This stage is generally split into two phases: the passive and the active, and the difference is dependent on whether you experience an urge or sensation to push your baby down and out or not.

Some women have an urge to push straight away and start the active phase immediately. For others, the sensation may take time to build, and this is absolutely fine. Your body will respond differently to other people's because you are different and that is part of what makes birth so beautiful.

Some women wish to be coached and encouraged to push while others prefer their body to guide them as to when and for how long to push. There is no right or wrong, it's just whatever feels best for you. If you have an epidural, then some guidance on pushing may be recommended as often you can't feel contractions or know when to push exactly (see Chapter 13 for more on pain relief).

As your baby descends, they push on the walls of the vagina, which stretches them. This, in turn, is sensed by your body, and signals are sent to the brain to secrete more oxytocin. The oxytocin causes more contractions, which encourages your baby down further.

As we touched on in Chapter 3, this positive feedback loop, helping you in this final stage, is called the Ferguson reflex and this creates a compulsive feeling and urge to push, similar to if you needed to have a poo. Pressure in your bottom is common as your baby moves low in the pelvis and is a great sign that things are progressing well.

A NOTE ON POOP AND BIRTH

I know that pooping during birth causes anxiety for many expectant mums (and it doesn't need to), so I want to offer some reassurance from the off. Doing a poo in labour is completely fine and normal: some people do it and some don't. Your midwife has seen everything (literally) before and will not be fazed in the slightest. Some women find they empty their bowels before active labour begins – as your uterus starts to get irritable and contract, it can cause you to go for a poo, in which case it is unlikely there will be any poo to come out later on anyway.

The reason why pooping can happen during birth is because the muscles you use when having a bowel movement are the same ones you engage when pushing in labour. There is also extra pressure on your colon and rectum when your baby moves through your birth canal and your baby is occupying lots of space, so if there is anything in your rectum (aka a poop), it is going to be pushed out. In fact, poop means your baby is descending ready to be born and that you are pushing with a great technique, so no midwife is ever going to be concerned about a poop in labour and neither should you be! Holding it in is only going to hold your baby in and that's pretty counterproductive, so go with it, and never worry about what your midwife thinks – what happens in the birth room stays in the birth room, sister!

As your baby's head becomes visible and continues to move down, this is called crowning. It is common for your baby to rock backwards and forwards in this stage as they are gently stretching the vaginal walls and perineum – baby's head may be visible with a contraction and then retreat back in between. This is your body naturally slowing down this stage to reduce the risk of tearing, and your baby is also navigating the curved section on your pelvis. This can feel frustrating, but keep in mind that, with each contraction, your baby comes a little bit further forward.

The head does one final stretch before being born and your midwife will encourage you to stop pushing and to breathe or blow, like a gentler version of your downwards breath, so that your baby's head is birthed as slowly as possible to continue to reduce the risk of tearing.

It is common to experience some sharp or burning pain as the tissues stretch for the final time, but this is very short-lasting and indicates that your baby's birth really is imminent. A warm compress can help soothe this stage. It is completely normal for there to be a pause for a couple of minutes between the birth of your baby's head and body, but don't worry as your baby is still getting oxygen from the placenta.

Every labour is different but, on average, once you start to push, you'll usually birth within one to three hours, although this can be much quicker if you've had a previous baby born vaginally. It is not recommended that this second, pushing stage of labour is too long, as a prolonged second stage can increase the chance of excessive bleeding post-birth, perineal tearing, infection or babies needing admission to intensive care. Your team will be supporting you to reduce the chances of all of these and making recommendations along the way to keep you and your baby safe and well.

I always encourage women to pause and appreciate what they have just achieved. So, when the time comes for you, I encourage you to pause and take it all in – it really is a momentous achievement.

You have crossed the bridge into motherhood: welcome to one of the most magical, life-affirming clubs there is.

THE THIRD STAGE

The third stage of labour is from after the birth of your baby to the delivery of your placenta.

The placenta is about the size of a small dinner plate and has been supplying your baby with nutrients and oxygen throughout pregnancy and removing their waste. It is connected to two different layers of membranes that create a sac (this is where your baby has been growing) and it is also connected to your baby's umbilical cord.

After your baby is born, the placenta peels away from the wall of your womb and is delivered through your vagina. This enables your uterus to shrink down and compress any exposed blood vessels from the placental site to control post-birth bleeding. Your uterus will then keep shrinking over the next six weeks or so back into your pelvis and to its pre-pregnancy size.

When your baby is born, they are still attached to your placenta by their umbilical cord until the cord is cut. This is a great opportunity to have delayed cord clamping, meaning the cord is not cut straight away, but that you and your team wait for 1–5 minutes so that your baby receives up to 30 per cent extra blood, as well as oxygen and stem cells through the cord first. There are lots of health benefits to your baby for this and it can happen whether they are preterm or full-term when they are born. Delayed cord clamping increases your baby's iron levels from birth and for as long as six months after birth too, supporting their development. It also increases the amount of stem cells your baby receives, which is an important factor in their immune system. There is massive benefit to leaving the cord for just one minute, but it can also be left longer if you wish. Delayed cord clamping can happen at all types of birth, including caesarean section birth. There may be some rare incidences when it cannot happen, but this is not commonplace and your team will explain why this was not possible.

There are generally two options for the delivery of your placenta, called active or physiological management. The active option involves an injection of a drug called syntocinon or syntometrine into your arm or leg muscle. This doesn't affect the ability to have delayed cord clamping or immediate skin-to-skin contact (see page 217). Your midwife will feel the cord to confirm it has stopped pulsating then clamp the cord and offer for you or your birthing partner to cut it. Then they will help to deliver your placenta by gently pressing on your tummy and applying some gentle traction in a downwards pulling motion on the umbilical cord to encourage the placenta out. This process may be mildly uncomfortable but shouldn't be painful. The other option is physiological management. This allows the oxytocin that is already in your body from labour to separate the placenta from your uterus naturally. The placenta is left to deliver with the aid of gravity and you pushing.

This stage generally takes 15–30 minutes, although physiological management may take up to 1 hour.

Active management is recommended by the National Institute for Health and Care Excellence (NICE) as it is has been shown to shorten the third stage of labour and reduce postpartum bleeding by 60 per cent. This also reduces the need for iron tablets or blood transfusions. This active option does result in a 1 per cent increase in the risk of nausea or vomiting due to the side effects of the medication used, though.

As with all aspects of your care, it is your choice and you do not have to decide until the time if you aren't sure. If there is an indication for active management to be strongly recommended to you to reduce your risk of excessive bleeding, such as a long labour, a medical condition or an instrumental birth, this will be discussed with you at the time.

Sometimes the placenta or part of the placenta or membranes can remain in the uterus, which is known as a retained placenta. This only happens in around 3 per cent of births and may need you to go to theatre to have it removed, in a procedure called a manual removal of the placenta, under regional anaesthesia such as a spinal anaesthetic.

This third stage provides a crucial bonding opportunity when your and your baby's hormone levels are at a peak and you have just been on the most powerful journey together, so I would recommend taking a moment to enjoy some precious, uninterrupted time, to embrace skin-to-skin and treasure meeting your baby after the journey you have been on. The golden hour is the hour immediately following your birth and is considered an optimal time to bond with and feed your baby. We will discuss the golden hour further in Chapter 17.

Bleeding after birth

One of the things that many of us picture about birth is blood. For the squeamish, this can be a concern, so having an idea about what to expect and why there is some bleeding after birth is helpful.

After your baby is born, the wound on your uterus where your placenta was attached will cause some bleeding, and there may also be some tears that can bleed. Bleeding is usually heaviest just after your baby is born and gradually becomes lighter over the next hours, days and weeks.

After the birth of your baby, blood loss will be weighed and calculated. A blood loss of up to 500ml is considered normal, while any loss over 500ml is considered a postpartum haemorrhage, though most women will not be affected by this. (It's worth noting that your body has prepared to lose some blood during birth through increasing your blood volume by around 50 per cent.) Don't worry, this isn't as much as it seems considering the average pregnant woman has around 5 litres of blood. Should you experience a postpartum haemorrhage, there is a lot the team can do to help you. This will usually involve medication and, in some rarer situations, a blood transfusion if you consent to this.

Boosting your iron stores in pregnancy is a really good idea to prevent anaemia and help you to recover from whatever degree of blood loss you may experience postnatally (see pages 71–2 for more on this).

The blood loss after the birth of your baby is called lochia and is made up of much more than just blood. It comprises blood, mucous, amniotic fluid, your baby's urine, skin cells and hair. Following birth, you continue to pass lochia, and the amount of blood lost and the length of time it continues for can vary considerably between women and is not necessarily dependent on the type of birth you have had. However, the average time is around two to four weeks.

Blood loss can start off heavy on the first day after you have your baby, so it's best to have some super absorbent pads at the ready. Blood loss is bright red initially, fading to pink or brown after a few days. You should keep an eye on your loss and seek medical advice if you notice that:

- you are regularly soaking through a maternity pad in less than two hours
- you are passing multiple clots or single large clots that are bigger than a golf ball
- you have persistent pain that doesn't go away or isn't relieved by simple painkillers such as paracetamol
- you feel ill, such as faint, dizzy, hot or sick

Remember, your body has cleverly adapted to tolerate bleeding post-birth and you have a team around you to ensure you are well looked after. It is best to avoid white underwear and have a good stash of maternity pads (these are chunkier than sanitary ones). It is recommended that pads are changed at least four-hourly, washing your hands before and after to help prevent infection.

YOUR ACTION PLAN TO BOSS EACH STAGE

Use your birth preference planner on page 226 to write down key, specific things you feel will help you through each stage of labour. You can refer back to this or ask your birth partner to when the time comes, and you will also find it useful to refer back to this plan once you have read further into Part 2.

The latent phase
For example, 'I will use my upwards breath, I will go for a walk, I will bake a cake . . .'

The first stage
For example, 'I will continue my upwards breath. I will adopt X, Y, Z positions. I will try X, Y, Z pain relief options (we'll cover positions and pain relief in Chapters 12 and 13). I will eat and drink X, Y, Z.'

The second stage
For example, 'I will use my downwards breath. I will use positive affirmations. I will ask my birth partner to do X, Y, Z when I am in transition stage . . .'

The third stage

For example, 'I will have immediate skin-to-skin. I will have delayed cord clamping. I will pause and look at my baby's X, Y, Z.'

Your labour really is a journey. Similar to that of pregnancy, there are distinct stages with different goals, each with a unique focus.

Next, we will look at the wonderful ways you may welcome your baby into the world.

REMEMBER:

- There are key stages to your labour journey. You know what your body and baby are trying to achieve and have a plan (above) on how you will manage each stage.
- You have more tools than you might realise to manage each stage of labour: breathing, mindset, pregnancy preparation and visualisations. We will build on these over the coming chapters too.
- Delayed cord clamping can take place in any birth and just one minute has huge positive impacts on your baby's health.

9

THE BEAUTIFUL WAYS YOU CAN BIRTH

No two births are the same – trust me, I have been in midwifery for over a decade and every single birth is unique. While you can prepare to influence your birth, there are some variables that are beyond your control and the exact way your birth plays out may well differ from what you planned. Through this chapter, we will explore all types of birth and I want you to be reassured that every birth can be positive and empowering regardless of the twists or turns that may crop up. I have also dedicated Chapter 10 to birth after a previous caesarean section. If you have not had a previous caesarean, you can skip this, but if you have, it will really help inform your options this time. I want to refer you back to a key message I spoke about in the introduction: a positive birth is not a certain *type* of birth, but, instead, it is a feeling.

The feeling of empowerment when you welcome
your baby into the world, however you may do so,
is where the secret to a positive birth lies.

I am dedicated to giving you no-stone-unturned, honest and comprehensive birth prep, and that is why we must make peace with the uncontrollable through this chapter. There will be some women who, despite the most diligent preparation, will birth by assisted vaginal or unplanned caesarean section. Here is the great news: these types of birth can be calm, empowering and truly positive experiences too.

> *Though there were many things I had little control over, I feel strong and powerful, even empowered, sore and full of love for how I birthed our daughter.*
>
> Rachel

UNASSISTED VAGINAL BIRTH

We are starting here because it is usually recommended to aim for an unassisted vaginal birth unless there is a medical reason why this would not be the safest option or you have made an informed decision to opt for a planned caesarean birth.

An unassisted vaginal birth is where your baby moves and navigates through your pelvis to reach your pelvic floor, passing under your pubic arch and through your vaginal canal to be born. You may have some medical support and intervention along the way, but your baby is born vaginally without the use of an instrument to help them out of the birth canal. The tips and information we have discussed to this point are directed at supporting your body to birth in this way: think of the optimal positioning of your baby (Chapter 4) and creating your oxytocin-promoting environment (Chapter 5) to assist your uterus to contract powerfully and regularly. We'll also look at positions for a better labour and birth in Chapter 12.

There are many benefits to an unassisted, vaginal birth, including a shorter hospital stay, a quicker recovery, lower risk of infections and lower risk of respiratory problems for your baby. It also reduces the likelihood of more significant perineal tearing and helps future pregnancies and births to be at lower risk of complication.

While you can follow all the tips and optimise your chances of an unassisted vaginal birth, sometimes birth may deviate from this path. It is important to be empowered with information about all modes of birth and to ensure you plan for how these can also be a positive experience.

Please remember there is no right or wrong, best or lesser way to birth your baby.

All birth is equal, and your birth is unique to you and your baby – there is a real beauty in the individual nature of birth, so let's embrace that and explore assisted vaginal birth.

ASSISTED VAGINAL BIRTH

Assisted vaginal birth is sometimes referred to as an 'instrumental birth' or an 'operative vaginal birth'. This type of birth involves an obstetrician using specifically designed instruments to help you to birth your baby vaginally.

Around 1 in 8 women in the UK has an assisted vaginal birth and this is increased to 1 in 3 first-time mums. These rates may be higher than you expected and that is why it is so important we talk about it so nothing is a surprise, and you can remain calm and confident as you welcome your little one earthside.

An assisted birth may be recommended if there are concerns over your or your baby's well-being, if pushing is not progressing as expected or if there is a medical condition that means you have been advised not to push during labour. Your obstetrician will explain the reasons for recommending assistance to you, along with the risks and benefits, and will answer any of your questions. They will ask to perform a VE with your consent to check that your cervix is fully dilated, to determine what position your baby is in and how low down in the birth canal they are. This enables your obstetrician to choose the best type of instrument for your individual situation to support your birth.

There are two types of instruments used with an assisted birth: the ventouse (also known as a kiwi or suction cup) or the forceps. These both work to assist with the physiological process of birth and both require you to still push your baby down, but they do have some key differences and one is likely to be more suitable for your situation over the other. The idea behind both is that they guide your baby down the birth canal as you push, and your baby's head should be born within two or three contractions.

The ventouse is a rubber or silicon cup that attaches to your baby's head using suction. During a contraction, you push and your obstetrician will gently pull to assist your baby's head out. Sometimes the cup may dislodge with a 'pop' sound and might need reapplying.

The forceps are smooth metal instruments that look like large spoons. They have a long handle, but only a small part actually sits in the vagina. They are designed in a curved shape in order to follow the natural curve of the birth canal and to cradle your baby's head. Often a forceps may be performed in a theatre instead and this is referred to as a 'trial'. This means that if, despite trying, your baby cannot be born vaginally, you are in the right place, with the right team, to proceed to a caesarean section.

There are some risks associated with assisted vaginal births that your obstetrician will discuss with you prior to you consenting to them, but here are some of the key ones to be aware of:

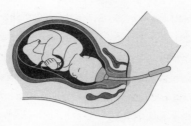

Ventouse birth

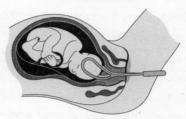

Forceps birth

- Bleeding can be heavier following birth with instrumental assistance, but your team will be keeping a close eye on this and have treatments and medication to control it.
- The chance of more extensive perineal tears is higher with the use of an instrument. The risk of third- and fourth-degree tears (see page 205) rises from 3 per cent to 4 per cent with the use of ventouse and 8–12 per cent with forceps. With a forceps birth, the instrument sits on the outside of the baby's head, so they increase the diameter that is coming out of your vagina. Because of this and to reduce the chance of these injuries, it is usually recommended to perform an episiotomy (a small cut into the perineum) to allow a little extra space for your baby to be born (see page 205).
- The chance of pelvic floor dysfunction and symptoms such as incontinence is higher. We have already discussed the pelvic floor in Chapter 4 and will delve into this again in Part 3 to help you know how to rehabilitate your pelvic floor post-birth to reduce dysfunction and symptoms.

- There may also be some marks on your baby's head that usually disappear in one to two days. These are usually very superficial and don't cause long-term issues. It is very rare to have any serious injury. In around 12 per cent of babies, the suction cup can cause a larger bruise that may result in jaundice in the first few days.
- A one-off dose of intravenous antibiotics is recommended following instrumental birth to reduce the chance of you developing an infection.

Your team will understand that an assisted vaginal birth is not your first choice of birth and that it can be anxiety-provoking. But remember, you can still have lots of your birth preferences: your birth bubble can still be maintained as well as having delayed cord clamping, skin-to-skin and your choice of music playing.

Often women will ask if it is best to have a caesarean section at this stage rather than an instrumental birth. However, a caesarean section in the final stages of labour can be more complicated, is associated with greater surgical risks and increases the chance of premature birth in future pregnancies and complications in future pregnancies. Although it is not always possible to avoid, it is usually not the first recommendation for this reason. However, do have a discussion with your obstetrician at the time to navigate the risks and benefits specific to your unique circumstance to help you make an informed decision.

Some women are able to take time to make these decisions depending on their circumstance and whether they are using pain relief, while for others these conversations can be more challenging as women can feel in a bit of a blur during labour. Your birth partner can help be part of these conversations and communicate things with you, although ultimately it will need to be you who makes the final choices as it is your body. It can also be beneficial to chat through some of the options 'just in case' at a time when you feel more able to take in your options and the information – having read and engaged with this book will also make this a smoother process for you as you are going in super informed.

Remember: it is your body. No one will do anything without your consent – you are always in charge.

I had a forceps birth with my little boy Jos. I had been in labour for quite a long time and, after having an epidural and starting to push, his heart rate was dropping and the doctor advised me that the best and quickest course of action would be to have a forceps birth with an episiotomy. I asked a number of questions, but ultimately put my trust in the medical team. I focused on my breathing and, after what seemed like seconds, he was in my arms. It was incredibly positive because even though I knew that I had got him so far, we needed a bit of help to get us to the finish line.

Beth

PLANNED OR UNPLANNED CAESAREAN BIRTH

Even if you are not planning a caesarean birth, it is a good idea to be informed about what a caesarean birth would look like for you. One in four women give birth by caesarean section, which means we are doing a huge injustice to 25 per cent of the motherhood population if we do not discuss this method of birth.

A note before we delve into caesarean birth: to undergo major abdominal surgery for the well-being of your baby to bring them safely earthside is one of the bravest, most courageous things you can do.

Caesarean birth mums are true warriors.

A caesarean section is an operation performed by an obstetrician where your baby is born through a cut in your abdomen. It involves a bikini line cut around 15cm long, just above your pubic hairline. It takes around ten minutes to enter the layers of your tummy, to stretch your abdominal muscles to the side and make a small cut on your uterus to reach your baby.

A caesarean section is usually performed under regional anaesthesia such as a spinal anaesthetic so that you can be awake at the birth of your baby, but occasionally, it may be necessary to perform a general anaesthetic – for example, if there is a medical reason why you cannot have a spinal anaesthetic, if the spinal anaesthetic is not working well enough or if there is serious concern over your baby's well-being and there is not time to allow a spinal anaesthetic to work. These situations are uncommon, and the aim is to have mothers awake to meet their baby whenever possible. If you are awake for a caesarean, then your birthing partner can be present with you and women will often report feeling some pushing or pulling sensations, but you should not feel any pain.

There are many reasons why a caesarean section may be performed, and they can be either a planned or elective procedure, or an unplanned emergency.

Some examples of planned caesarean section reasons include a baby in a breech position, a previous caesarean section, a placenta praevia (where your placenta covers your cervix and labour is contraindicated) or for maternal request.

Some examples of why an unplanned or emergency caesarean section may be recommended are if labour is not progressing as expected, if there are concerns about a mother's or baby's well-being, such as infection, significant bleeding or if a baby becomes distressed in labour.

Caesarean sections are broken down into four categories depending on the reason:

- Category 1: Concern over immediate threat to life, should be performed as soon as possible and within 30 minutes.
- Category 2: Concern over compromise to mother or baby, but not immediately life-threatening. Birth to be within 75 minutes.
- Category 3: No compromise to mother or baby but early birth is needed.
- Category 4: Birth is timed to suit woman and healthcare provider – planned or elective caesarean sections.

A caesarean section is generally a safe procedure but, as with any surgery, there are risks and possible complications, including risks associated with a subsequent pregnancy after having had a caesarean section. Your obstetrician will discuss these with you at the time specific to your individual circumstance should a caesarean be recommended and will take your informed consent for the procedure.

Generally, the stitches used are all dissolvable. You will have a catheter in your bladder for around 12 hours as you will not have full sensation in your legs or bladder for a little while after and women will typically stay in hospital for one to two nights after birth. The recovery with a caesarean birth is slower than a vaginal birth and you will need some extra assistance as you recover. Recovery time frames are very different for each woman – everyone's recovery journey is unique. It is worth checking with your insurance company if you drive as many do not cover you for the six weeks after surgery. It is recommended to avoid driving and heavy lifting in this time, but gentle and early mobilisation and staying on top of your painkillers is recommended.

During a caesarean section (or when an assisted vaginal birth is performed in theatre), there are quite a few people in theatre. Sometimes this many people can feel overwhelming, but try to remember they all have a role to play in keeping you and your baby safe. You have a room full of experts looking after you and that can be really reassuring.

So how can you make a caesarean birth a calm and positive experience? Caesarean birth has come a long way in recent years. It need not be viewed as a clinical surgical procedure and can instead be an individualised, empowering and positive way of giving birth considering your birth preferences and choices.

The term 'gentle caesarean birth' is becoming more familiar. A gentle caesarean makes the experience feel like the birthing experience that it is and allows aspects of a vaginal birth to be incorporated. There is no one set way to have a gentle caesarean as the wishes of each family will vary just as they do during a vaginal birth, but the principles can usually be applied for both planned and unplanned caesarean births:

- Delayed cord clamping (see page 127): in just one minute your baby receives around 30 per cent extra blood volume, which has a whole heap of health benefits for them.
- Immediate, or as soon as possible, skin-to-skin contact: your team may be able to arrange drapes in such a way that you can have immediate skin-to-skin during delayed cord clamping without impacting the sterile environment. If this is not possible, skin-to-skin once the cord is cut before any routine checks can be facilitated. Most babies born by caesarean section do not need any immediate care, but for those who do

there will be a skilled team ready to support them. They will keep you updated and will get you to see, touch and hold your baby as soon as possible.

- Dropping of the drapes: as your baby is born the surgical drapes can be dropped so that you and your birth partner can see the special moment that your baby is brought into the world. Some women may hold a mirror to see their birth clearer.

- A calm environment: you may be birthing in theatre, but it can still feel like a relaxing and positive space. Mood and/or dim lighting, an eye mask to block any bright lights, your choice of music playing and the presence of your birth partner can all make a really big impact on the whole experience.

- You can take your camera into theatre to capture those magical first moments as your little one is welcomed earthside.

- Although not always possible, some women choose to provide time for their baby to 'walk' out of the caesarean incision in a gentler way than a surgeon guiding them out with their hands. This is generally safer in a planned than unplanned caesarean birth where there may be more haste needed for a baby to be born.

Remember, this is your birth, your body and your baby. You are the birth boss, and you are in control. It is useful to communicate your preferences around an abdominal birth with your team should it be recommended to you.

However you birth your baby, you are a real-life superwoman.

The goal for my C-section was to feel connected with the experience and part of the process, not just witness it. For me, this meant thinking about why I considered a vaginal birth to be the most natural of births and, from this, how the 'natural' elements could be worked into the operation.

This began with a calm, quiet theatre. I kindly requested for no 'water cooler'-style chat to happen over my head. I wanted to be able to ask questions without interrupting and to hear the first tiny squeaks, muffles or cries of my baby, not what the medical staff were having for lunch.

For background noise we had a playlist and the song 'Today' that was playing when they lifted my son earthside is as memorable to us as our first dance song.

Lighting was similarly important to me. I feel at ease when the lights are low so I requested for all non-essential lighting to be turned off or dimmed and to have natural light where possible.

With the scene set, it was time to think about the actual birth. Witnessing my baby entering the world was a top priority, so I requested for the screen to be dropped and, if possible, for my baby to be 'walked out' of the womb. I wanted him to enter slowly, being squeezed in the process – like babies do when they travel through the birth canal – rather than being taken from the womb and held up like Simba from The Lion King *under bright lights.*

Although this birth was clinical, it was calm and I felt I had as much control as medically possible. There wasn't a birthing pool and fairy lights, but there was oxytocin by the bucket load and that, for me, was everything.

Amy

TWINS, TRIPLETS AND MULTIPLES

Multiple pregnancies are on the rise. Interestingly, in 1984 only 1 in 100 births were multiples and now it is around 1 in every 65.

The first note here is that, while every pregnancy is super unique and individual, this is the case even more so with multiples, so your antenatal appointments and scans will be important in supporting you through your birth choices.

With multiple pregnancies there are some key differences to be aware of and to factor into your birth preference planning. For example, around 60 per cent of twins and 75 per cent of triplets are born preterm and, depending on how early babies are born, how big they are and how well they adapt to being in the outside world, they may require some care in the neonatal intensive care unit (NICU) for a period of time. I would therefore recommend reading Chapter 17.

You may have already noticed that your pregnancy is being kept a super close eye on with regular appointments, and this will also be the case when it comes to planning for birth. Depending on your individual circumstances, you may be recommended to birth by planned caesarean section or to have an earlier induction of labour than someone with just one baby. The rationale for these recommendations should be explained to you by your obstetrician, but if you do feel unsure of the reason, I would recommend using the BRAIN tool (see page 98) to help you understand and make informed decisions. If you are having a vaginal birth with multiples, the recommendation is to birth on a labour ward and to have your babies' heart rates continuously monitored during labour to keep a close eye on how they are managing the process.

One of the most helpful things for women expecting multiples is to hear from those who have been through multiple births themselves, so let me share these words of wisdom from Kate Ball @ noahsarkfamily, founder of Mini First Aid @minifirstaid (see Further Resources, page 311) and the super mum of not one, but two sets of twins . . .

I'm Kate Ball, mum of six (two singletons and two sets of non-identical twins). I found out I was pregnant with my second set of twins when my first set had just turned one! Both sets born just 20 months apart!

Here are my top tips for twin (and multiples) pregnancy.

Doctors and midwives need to review and monitor twin pregnancies closely and regularly, so be prepared for more frequent scans and appointments. It's worth telling your employer too as you may need to take more time off work for appointments than a typical singleton pregnancy.

There is often complicated terminology used in twin and multiple pregnancies, the type you have, how the babies are lying in the womb, etc. — if you don't understand, ask! You need to be confident that you absolutely understand and don't get lost in medical terminology.

Be kind to your body — growing multiple babies at the same time can put added pressure on your back, knees, ankles and pelvic area. I survived with pregnancy Pilates, regular massage and accepting that my feet needed to be up a lot!

Twins are often smaller in birth weight, which means they need teeny clothes. The hospitals will always support to start with if you are short of outfits for the babies, but it's a good idea to be prepared with some preemie-size baby clothes.

I had a really good birth plan with my midwife, but it's important to have an open mind. Sometimes plans have to change for the safety of you and your babies, and often more medical professionals need to be present for delivery. Prepare yourself to be open to a change of birth plan, and get your birth partner to advocate for you, ask questions and make sure that you can stay calm. There is no 'best way' for babies to be born. The priority is you and your babies.

Twin and multiple pregnancies are often shorter than a typical singleton pregnancy (births before 37 weeks). Get prepared at home early so that you don't get caught out. After a twin delivery, you and your babies may also have to have a longer stay in hospital. It's good to be prepared for a longer stay, with all the extra bits and pieces, and be mentally prepared so that you are not disappointed and stressed.

I recommend joining the Twins Trust (see Further Resources, page 311) – there is a multitude of really good advice for both pregnancy and beyond and discounts for buying everything you need. (I write a regular column in their magazine too!)

As the founder of Mini First Aid, I would recommend that EVERY expectant parent learns baby first aid – it's a must and will give you the peace of mind you deserve.

And don't forget that you will need lots of nappies – lots and lots!

PAUSE FOR THOUGHT

One of the key things to do in ensuring your birth is a positive experience is to plan for your least-preferable type and then recognise how you can add your stamp to it, implement some of the things that are transferable and feel really important to you to ultimately shape it more positively. This may also flag some questions around specific types of birth you wish to ask your care provider about at your next appointment – jot these down on paper or in your phone now so you have them to hand.

- What type of birth feels least-preferable to you?
- How can you create positive feelings, calm emotions and empowerment within this? Reading the birth stories may help you with ideas here (scan the QR code on page 6).
- Do you have any questions based on this to ask your midwife or obstetrician?

The next chapter is dedicated to those who have had a previous caesarean section birth.

REMEMBER:

- All birth is equal – there is no one way better than the other, and it can all be equally empowering and positive.
- Plan for all types of birth. Being informed of the twists and turns that birth can take is a powerful way of helping you be calm and in control.
- Know that, in the vast majority of births, even when it has been labelled an emergency, there is usually time for you to ask a question or express something that is important to you.

10

BIRTHING AFTER A PREVIOUS CAESAREAN SECTION

There are lots of mums who have had a previous caesarean section and are wondering what that means for future birth. If this is you, I have written this chapter to ensure that you are well-equipped to navigate your options and make informed choices about your birth. I have included a lot of detail here for you because, in my mind, mums don't get the degree of information they need or deserve to make an informed choice. If this chapter isn't relevant to you, please do skip on to Chapter 11.

Please also know that if your previous birth was a traumatic experience or you have some questions you would like answers to, there are birth reflection or debriefing services available, so speak with your community midwife so you can be booked into one.

YOUR OPTIONS AFTER A PREVIOUS CAESAREAN SECTION

If you have had a previous caesarean birth, you generally have two options for your future birth: a vaginal birth after caesarean section (VBAC) or a planned or elective repeat caesarean section birth (ERCS). Let's take a moment to look at these two options in more detail.

Vaginal Birth After Caesarean Section (VBAC)

VBAC is the term used for women who have had a previous caesarean section and wish to have a vaginal birth in a subsequent pregnancy.

If you are planning a VBAC, it is usually best to aim to go into spontaneous labour because this has the highest rate of VBAC success. All the tips and tricks discussed throughout Parts 1 and 2 will help you in this. But it is also important to try not to feel that 'due date pressure' I talked about in Chapter 4 (page 74) because, remember, your baby is the biggest influence in deciding when labour will begin.

Around your due date, your obstetrician may wish to discuss options with you if you have not yet gone into labour and these will likely be: continuing to wait for labour to start, induction of labour or an ERCS (see page 151). Bring your decision-making tools from Chapter 6 to the forefront here and know from all the birth planning you are doing that, whichever way you welcome your baby into your arms, you will be incredible.

If you are planning a VBAC birth and you go into labour, you should feel a sense of calm confidence that your body and baby are on a great path. It is usually recommended to birth on a delivery suite or labour ward where there's access to a medical team and theatre. Your contractions and baby can then be closely monitored and you will have all the medical professionals to hand in case you need their support. Some women may wish to have their VBAC outside of these guidelines, such as in a birthing centre or at home, and your team will always support your wishes. But it is important to have a detailed conversation ahead of time about all the options, so, if you feel you may like to talk through something that is different to standard guidance, it is best to mention this as early on as possible.

The pros and cons specific to your individual circumstance should be talked through with your obstetrician to allow you to make an informed choice on your care. An individual care plan can then be made for you so that, when you do go into labour, all the staff that are on call know what your wishes are, how they can support you and that you have already been well- informed.

I was empowered to ask questions and make plans that were tailored to me, even when this wasn't following exactly what the hospital recommended. In the end I didn't get my VBAC, but I felt so powerful even though there was so much I couldn't control. I was in a much better place for having thoroughly prepared.

Rachel

Elective Repeat Caesarean Section (ERCS)

If you have decided that you wish to birth through an ERCS, you may be wondering when it will be scheduled for. The answer is usually 39 weeks. The reason for this is, prior to being born, your baby doesn't use their lungs to breathe because the placenta provides them with all the oxygen they need, so during pregnancy their lungs are full of fluid instead of air. In the later stages of pregnancy, your baby's lungs start absorbing some of this fluid, then in labour, through contractions and as baby passes though the vaginal canal, even more fluid is squeezed out. When a baby is born and they take their first breath, their lungs fill up with air and more fluid is pushed out. Any leftover fluid is slowly absorbed through their bloodstream and lymphatic system or coughed out. Babies with a condition called transient tachypnea of the newborn (TTN) have too much fluid still in their lungs when they are born, which means they have to work harder at breathing and breathe faster to get enough oxygen into their lungs. This may mean they have a short stay in the NICU to support them with this transition. As TTN risk is less after 39 weeks and planned caesarean section is a known risk factor for TTN because your baby doesn't have any of that squeezing from contractions (see page 124), ERCS without other complication is usually scheduled in your 39th week of pregnancy.

Naturally, women who are opting for an ERCS may feel concern about going into labour prior to their planned date. If this does happen, your caesarean section will be performed sooner and classed as an emergency caesarean section (EMCS), although some women may decide to try for a VBAC if labour starts spontaneously and is progressing smoothly. It is your choice, and your team will support you in this.

DECIDING WHAT IS RIGHT FOR YOU

Making the decision on whether to choose a VBAC or ERCS can feel overwhelming at first if you don't have strong gut feelings towards one option or the other. Looking through the individual circumstances of you and your baby with your midwife and obstetrician is important in ensuring you have all the pieces of the puzzle to make an informed choice.

'I am strong enough to let my baby be born the way baby needs.'

There are some key considerations and questions I recommend discussing with your obstetrician and midwife which will assist you in your decision-making and will allow the statistics and evidence to feel more relevant to you and your circumstances:

- **Why did you have a previous caesarean section?** VBAC success rates vary depending on the reason for a previous caesarean section. Your obstetrician will look at your previous labour and surgery notes to gain more information on this for you.

- **Were there any complications?** This may give more information as to how your labour may go this time and how your scar may cope with contractions.
- **What type of incision did you have?** Most caesarean section incisions are done as a horizontal, lower-segment incision on your 'bikini line', but occasionally they may be done vertically, called a 'classical' incision, and this is associated with more complications in future pregnancy.
- **How do you feel about your previous labour and birth experience?** If there are certain elements that have caused birth trauma or anxiety, your team can refer you for counselling and put measures in place to help ensure things are more positive for you this time round. If you feel you are navigating some existing trauma from your previous birth, please contact the Birth Trauma Association (Further Resources, page 311) where you can be supported and signposted to help.
- **How many previous caesarean sections have you had?** This has an impact on the risks and success rate of a VBAC.
- **Have you had any previous vaginal births?** Women who have had a previous vaginal birth tend to have a higher VBAC success rate.
- **How many children do you wish to have?** Caesarean section risk increases with each caesarean section, so this is a consideration if you are planning many more children.

Although ideally you may decide by 36 weeks, please remember there is no rush and you may change your mind and wish to revisit the discussion at a later date, and that is fine too.

There are some benefits and risks to all modes of birth and, when deciding about an ERCS or a VBAC, it is useful to look at these with the Scales tool we discussed in Chapter 6 (see page 97).

Note down where you feel the pros and cons sit for you as I go through the evidence below (there is a table on page 158 to help you with this).

Generally speaking, after one previous caesarean section around 75 per cent of women who have a straightforward pregnancy and who go into labour spontaneously (without induction of labour) will have a successful VBAC. If you have had a previous vaginal birth, this increases to an 80–90 per cent chance of a successful VBAC.

There are some circumstances when a VBAC may not be recommended for you and these include: women who have had more than three previous caesarean births, if you have had a previous uterine rupture or a previous classical caesarean incision, or if you have had any other pregnancy complication that requires a planned caesarean birth.

The likelihood of a successful VBAC has also been linked to the reason for the previous caesarean section and this can generally be divided into two categories: recurrent and non-recurrent reasons. What this is essentially looking at is how likely it is that the same issue will arise again and therefore the chance that the same complication will result in another unplanned caesarean section. Recurrent (more likely to happen again) reasons included: slow progress in labour, prolonged second stage of labour, unsuccessful induction of labour and macrocosmic (big) baby. Non-recurrent (less likely to happen again) reasons included: distress of baby in labour, malpresentation (where your baby is not in an optimal head-down position), such as breech or transverse lie, or placenta praevia (see page 141). The VBAC success rates for those with a recurrent factor was around 50–67 per cent, compared to closer to 89 per cent for those with a non-recurrent reason for previous caesarean section.

Now you understand the options available to you, it is time to break it all down into the advantages and disadvantages of each option. Remember to use the table on page 158 to jot down the pros and cons of each option that feel most prominent to you as an individual, bearing in mind the Scales tool from Chapter 6, to help you make informed decisions.

Pros of VBAC:

- The recovery and hospital stay following a vaginal birth is quicker than that following a caesarean section birth.
- Vaginal birth is more often associated with lower bleeding and infection rates than caesarean birth.
- You avoid the risks of surgery by having a VBAC and reduce complications in future pregnancy or birth.

Cons of VBAC:

- There is always a risk of needing an unplanned caesarean section or EMCS – this happens in around 25 per cent of women. This is a slight increase to the risk of EMCS in women labouring for the first time without having had a previous caesarean section, where the risk is around 20 per cent.
- An EMCS carries higher levels of surgical risk than an elective/planned caesarean section (ELCS) as the circumstances are usually more time-pressured and the surgery may be more complicated in different stages of labour.
- You have a slightly higher chance of needing a blood transfusion than women who birth by ELCS.
- There is a 1 in 200 (0.5 per cent) risk of the scar on your uterus tearing/opening during labour – this is termed 'scar rupture'. If your labour is induced, this risk

increases to 1–1.5 per cent. If this complication was suspected or confirmed, an EMCS would be recommended immediately.

- You may require an assisted vaginal birth using ventouse or forceps (see page 135) and may sustain perineal injury or tearing (as with a vaginal birth without previous caesarean section).
- Serious complications to baby such as stillbirth or brain injuries are the same as for any woman labouring for the first time, but are higher than with an ELCS.

Pros of ERCS:

- The risk of uterine rupture is lower at 0.1 per cent.
- The risks of labour and rare, serious complications for baby are lower at 0.2 per cent.
- You will have a known date for your ERCS birth, although this can be subject to change, and around 1 in 10 women go into labour prior to this date, which is usually around 39 weeks.
- No perineal tearing.
- May help you feel more in control, which can be important if you have experienced previous birth trauma.

Cons of ERCS:

- Caesarean sections are major abdominal surgical procedures that carry risks of surgery and longer recovery and healing times. A repeat caesarean section may take longer and be more difficult than the first due to the presence of scar tissue.
- You may have a longer recovery period than with a VBAC and may need additional help at home. You will

be unable to drive for six weeks post-birth (it's worth checking this with your insurance company).

- Caesarean sections carry a risk of damage to surrounding structures such as the bladder or bowel.

- The risk of excessive bleeding and requiring a blood transfusion is higher.

- There is a risk of infection to the wound which causes complications with healing. Your team will advise you if you are at higher risk of infection such as if you have a raised body mass index (see page 167), diabetes or there was a surgical complication.

- You have a higher chance of thrombosis with a caesarean section, which is where blood clots develop in the legs (deep vein thrombosis) or in the lungs (pulmonary embolism), and you may therefore be recommended anti-thrombotic injections to reduce this risk.

- If planning further pregnancies, you will be more likely to need another caesarean section, which results in further scar tissue and increases the chance of your placenta growing abnormally and into the previous scar tissues. This is called placenta accreta or percreta and they are termed 'abnormally invasive placentas'. These placentas are rare, but are more complicated to remove in future births, which means bleeding can be heavier and there is a higher chance of hysterectomy (uterus being removed).

- In 2 per cent of caesarean section births the baby's skin may accidentally be cut, though this usually heals well without complication.

- Babies born by caesarean section have an increased risk of breathing problems. However, this typically doesn't last too long and is the main reason why ERCS is not recommended before 39 weeks. Babies born without labour are at a higher risk of breathing complications such as TTN, as they do not clear lung fluid in the way a baby does who has had the impact of contractions and/or a vaginal birth. Four to five per cent of babies born by ERCS after 39 weeks have breathing problems compared to 2–3 per cent born by VBAC. If an ERCS is performed at 38 weeks, the risk increases to 6 per cent.

	VBAC	ERCS
Pros:		
Cons:		

VBAC or ERCS is such a unique decision and I hope this chapter will help guide you in making the right choice for you.

The next chapter is all about helping you understand induction of labour and how this can be a positive birth experience.

REMEMBER:

- You and your baby are individuals and there are many factors that may influence your future birth plans. Have open conversations with your care provider so they can best support you.

- If you are planning a VBAC, it is a sensible approach to also consider what a positive ERCS would look like for you so that you ultimately have a positive experience either way.

- It is useful to think about what you may like to happen if you plan an ERCS and your body goes into labour. You could have an EMCS or a VBAC if there are no contraindications to vaginal birth for you.

11

INDUCING LABOUR

I have chosen to dedicate a whole chapter to the induction of labour because it is a big topic with lots of ifs, buts and maybes, and is an area that lots of the women I meet don't have the amount of knowledge on that they deserve. My mission through this chapter is to make sure that this is not the case for you. In 2010, in England 21 per cent of labours were induced. By March 2021 this had risen to 34 per cent, meaning that 1 in 3 women have an induction of labour. This is the reason why we must talk about induction of labour to understand it, be empowered and prepared. It is important to remember that induction of labour is not something to fear. There are often many negative stories around it, which feeds into the birth-fear culture that is so damaging to your physiological birth hormones.

In this chapter, I will guide you through common reasons for induction, why induction may be offered to you, how to navigate your options and how to make informed decisions. If you do decide that an induction of labour is the best option for you and your baby, I will then discuss the tools and techniques you need to have a positive induction of labour experience and an empowered birth.

I was very worried about being induced at first as I was told that induction can be lengthy, especially for the first baby. I even cried when I was told that I'd need to be induced, because I didn't know what to expect.

I was induced at 3pm on the Saturday and I was expecting it to be a slow process. My husband went home and only got one hour of sleep as, at 1am Sunday, my waters broke. An hour later I was moved to the labour ward and our baby was born at 6:46am! Only five hours of labour for my first baby after being induced.

I had the most positive birth and the induction was a very fast process for me. I wish I'd never listened to all the horror stories people told me about induction and ending in C-sections, as this was far from the reality for me.

Annabel

ESTIMATED DUE DATES

Before we delve into induction of labour, we need to address the term 'due date'. In the UK, following your 12-week ultrasound scan, you are given an estimated due date of 40 weeks. But here is the thing: only around 5 per cent of babies are born on this date, which means we must highlight the term 'estimated'.

I encourage you to consider a window where birth is likely rather than a particular date, because it is highly likely that your little one will not show up on this date and, despite your best efforts, it is easy to fall into the trap of 'due date pressure'. Be mindful also of who you tell about your estimated due date; there is nothing more frustrating when trying to calmly, patiently await your baby's arrival than a pinging phone with well-meaning (or nosey) friends and family asking about your pending birth.

Let's be honest, we are all much too unique to have the same gestational period – our furry dog pals have a super short gestation of just two months whereas poor elephants are pregnant for almost two years. Even within humans, the global use of a 'due date' is not consistent, highlighting how we simply do not know (and never will) what date is the perfect date for you and your baby. As I mentioned in Chapter 4, there is increasing evidence to suggest that the baby triggers the onset of labour when they are ready by sending chemical signals to the mother's hormonal system. This triggers prostaglandin release, and this hormonal dance between mother and baby is what causes labour to begin.

Given that around 80 per cent of first-time mums-to-be will still be pregnant as they watch their due date come and go, this realistic expectation around a due date is really important to consider. If we look at a 'due window' instead, then we need to understand that, in the UK, 37–42 weeks is considered full-term.

REASONS FOR INDUCTION OF LABOUR

Induction may be offered to you for a variety of reasons, including medical conditions, if your waters break (but labour does not follow over the next 24 hours), concerns over the well-being of mother or baby, or going 'overdue'. An induction, like all medical interventions, may be offered to you if your obstetrician feels the benefits outweigh the risks of the pregnancy continuing for you or your baby depending on the specific reason. The rationale, risks, benefits or alternatives specific to you should be discussed with you at the time so that you can make an informed decision.

The BRAIN tool we discussed in Chapter 6 is an ideal tool to use when looking at your options around induction of labour. Below is an example of the BRAIN tool in action. I used this myself in pregnancy as, as my mum had long pregnancies, I assumed I would be the same. It turns out I wasn't and my son was born fashionably late two days after his estimated due date (which, as a side note, is a good reason to not allow experiences of family members to make you feel your birth will follow the same path).

USING THE BRAIN TOOL FOR INDUCTION OF LABOUR

- Benefits: May reduce the chance of stillbirth if I do not go into labour spontaneously by 42 weeks.
- Risks: May be a long process, which means staying in hospital. May be more uncomfortable through additional examinations and induction medication. Induction medication may cause too many contractions (hyperstimulation – see page 174).
- Alternatives: I will be offered induction from 41 weeks, as my pregnancy hasn't had any complications. I could keep a close eye on my baby's movements for a couple of extra days, try a stretch and sweep and see if I go into labour.
- Intuition: I feel comfortable waiting until 41+3, but if I have any concerns over my baby's well-being I will call the hospital sooner.
- Nothing: I could continue without any additional monitoring or induction.

Just writing down and formulating my thoughts like this as I approached my due date was reassuring. Perhaps the comfort of having done this exercise is what helped my labour start on its own before induction was even offered . . . who knows? What is important here is to know that your BRAIN will look different to mine – we are individual so two will never be the same, but I hope seeing it in action helps you to use it too.

I feel it is important that we are transparent around the current evidence base in relation to induction of labour. The reality is it is not possible to always gain high-quality evidence in pregnancy and birth outcomes as it would simply not be ethical to conduct the research. As a result, this can make some decisions around your options such as induction of labour feel a little tricky.

Below are some of the common reasons for offering induction of labour. It is important to highlight, however, that we are all individual and may have other influences in our medical or pregnancy history that are more complex than this page can cover, so having a conversation with your obstetrician or midwife is important when making your decision about induction.

Postdates or 'overdue'

One of the most common reasons for being offered an induction of labour is going 'overdue'. The stats show that 82.8 per cent of labours start spontaneously by 40+6 weeks and 99 per cent by 41+6 weeks of pregnancy. If you have had an uncomplicated pregnancy, then you may be offered an induction of labour between 41 and 42 weeks (7–14 days past your due date). The rationale for this is that, beyond 42 weeks, there is an increase in the risk of stillbirth. This is where I always encourage expectant parents to examine the numbers and statistics (as discussed in Chapter 6); at 37 weeks the risk of stillbirth is 1 in every 3,000 births, rising to 6 in every 3,000 births after 43 weeks.

'Small' baby

A 'small' baby may be small for many different reasons: from your genetics, and it therefore being a very normal size for them, to a restriction in their growth. If it is suspected that your baby's growth is restricted, this could be because your placenta is not working as well as it should and therefore you may be offered an induction of labour.

'Big' baby

The medical terminology for a big baby is 'macrosomia'. There is some difficultly around determining accurate estimates of baby's size during pregnancy as ultrasound scans in the UK are 85 per cent accurate, meaning your baby's size could be 15 per cent larger or smaller than the estimated size on a scan. Don't get me wrong here, scans are a fantastic resource and sonographers who perform them are experts, but the nature of the process means they are not 100 per cent accurate and there is always a margin for error. It is important that there is total transparency about this when making decisions based upon the findings, especially when looking at size alone.

The worry around a suspected 'big' baby is the chance of a birth complication known as a shoulder dystocia. This is when there is difficulty with baby's shoulders being born and happens in around 1 in 150 births. There has been a recent review to look at whether induction of labour may help to reduce the chance of shoulder dystocia and problems for mums and babies when the baby is suspected to be larger. The study found that shoulder dystocia was reduced by approximately 27 per 1,000 babies when labour was induced, and third- and fourth-degree tears (see page 205) were reduced by 19 per 1,000 women. There was no difference in caesarean birth or instrumental birth rates between the induced or non-induced groups. While an induction may have pros in such situations, induction itself comes with some cons too which we will discuss on page 173.

Advanced maternal age

The risk of stillbirth is low in older mothers, but there is an increase in this risk for women over the age of 40 years and the reason for this is largely unknown. At 39–40 weeks of pregnancy, the risk of stillbirth in a mother over 40 years is 2 in 1,000 compared to 1 in 1,000 for women under 35. Women over 40 years of age at 39 weeks have a similar stillbirth risk to women in their mid-twenties at 41 weeks. Based on this evidence, induction of labour is usually offered to women aged over 40 years from 39 weeks of pregnancy.

IVF pregnancy

There is research suggesting that stillbirth rates are increased for babies conceived through IVF treatment. A Danish study showed a rate increase from 3.7 per 1,000 babies to 16.2 per 1,000 babies. Based on this, induction of labour is commonly offered for IVF pregnancy.

Gestational diabetes

There are lots of variables within gestational diabetes, but higher blood sugar levels may lead to a bigger than average baby, birth complications and an increased risk of stillbirth. The better blood sugar control is the lower these risks become and, depending on your gestational diabetes and individual circumstance, you may be offered induction of labour.

Raised body mass index (BMI)

Some women may be offered induction of labour based on a raised BMI in pregnancy. This should be discussed on an individual basis as the evidence is not clear.

The topic of BMI and weight in pregnancy can feel challenging to discuss. I'd therefore like to share with you some advice from Dr Alice Keely, known as The Heavyweight Midwife, as she specialises in supporting women with plus-size pregnancy:

Many pregnant plus-size women worry about their weight in pregnancy for two reasons: whether their weight will affect their health, their pregnancy and their baby; and how they will be treated by doctors and midwives.

The truth is that complications are unlikely for any woman of any size. This is true for plus-size women – the chances of complications are a bit higher, but they are still low. Your weight during pregnancy is a consideration for your care and your plans, not a complication in itself. There are some extra tests and scans that might be recommended, but if you do not experience complications, there is no reason why you should be treated any differently for labour and birth. Try to be open with your midwife – tell them if you are worried about how you'll be treated because of your weight. That way you're explicitly asking them for support.

If you are nervous for your appointments and scans, make sure you write down questions, take a support person, ask the questions and take notes. And if a health professional says you are 'high risk', ask them to be a bit more specific, say, how many women in every 100 would experience that complication, for example. Similarly, if anyone says your risk is 'doubled', ask for actual numbers (for example, your risk of developing gestational diabetes is 'doubled' in pregnancy if you are plus size, but around 90 per cent of plus-size women do not get gestational diabetes).

Remember that dieting in pregnancy is not known to be safe, but also NHS advice on healthy eating and weighing women in pregnancy does not consider the many women who have an eating disorder or have had one in the past, and this is of concern and needs attention and research. Health is holistic – it is about eating well, sleeping well, exercising and looking after your mind as well as your body.

I have covered just some of the common reasons induction is offered here. I always encourage you to evaluate the numbers whenever considering risk, but to also recognise that you and your baby are not as simple as a number; you are human beings with a whole different set of circumstances and needs.

My induction of labour was so empowering, primal and magical, and I would do it all over again in a heartbeat!

Abi

STRETCH AND SWEEPS

A stretch and sweep may be offered to you around your due date by your midwife and it can be considered a form of induction, albeit without any medication being involved. You may be familiar with this term already, but I want to share some more information with you so that you understand it comprehensively, can have a think about whether it may be something you wish to try and, ultimately, to ensure it is not something you feel worried about.

A stretch and sweep is an internal VE where your midwife will try to put one or two fingers into your cervix, sweeping their finger around the cervix to try to gently wriggle or 'sweep' the membranes from your cervix, creating some stimulation. The aim is to encourage the release of hormones called prostaglandins that are responsible for the softening and ripening of the cervix.

As you are now learning, there are potential risks and benefits to all interventions, so let's examine what those may look like for a stretch and sweep so you can make an informed decision and feel in control.

Possible benefits of a stretch and sweep:

- Reduced chance of medical induction in 75 per cent of first-time mums and 80 per cent of mums who have given birth before.

- 79 per cent of women will go into labour within seven days of a stretch and sweep.
- Decreased length of pregnancy by 1–4 days.

Possible risks of a stretch and sweep:

- Vaginal bleeding.
- Pain/discomfort when being performed.
- Unable to perform if the cervix is closed.
- Stop-and-start latent phase of labour (the earliest part of labour we talked through in Chapter 8).
- A 9 per cent chance of breaking waters unintentionally if a stretch and sweep is performed during labour.

The key challenge with a stretch and sweep is that we will never be sure if it caused a woman to go into labour or if she was going to labour anyway and we just so happened to do one. Some women swear by them working for them, others want to give it a go in case it works and, for others, it feels like a form of intervention they wish to avoid. There is no black and white and definitely no right or wrong here. You will be supported to do what you feel is best for you and your baby after talking through your options and all the pros and cons with your healthcare practitioner.

WHAT HAPPENS DURING AN INDUCTION OF LABOUR

An induction aims to mirror the same processes we discussed in Chapter 8 for labour: the latent stage, the first stage and the second stage (see page 113). The exact way your labour may be induced varies depending on the hospital you receive care from, as they have different policies. Your individual medical and pregnancy history will also influence the way your labour is induced, as there are different ways to do it.

The first step is to soften your cervix, which is what happens in the latent phase of labour. This may be done in a variety of ways, and it is a useful idea to check in with your midwife about the method they use so you know what that could look like for you should you be offered it.

I am going to give you a little overview of the different methods used here so that, no matter which your hospital uses, you are familiar with what they involve:

- **Prostaglandin pessaries or gels:** These are inserted vaginally and may be a slow-release pessary or gel tablets. During this stage you will be able to walk around and eat and drink as normal. Most hospitals require you to stay in as an inpatient for the duration of the induction process. The pessary or gel will remain in for a period of time, usually between 6 and 24 hours. Your cervix is then re-examined to see if it has opened enough for your waters to be broken. Repeat doses may also be given if needed.
- **Mechanical induction:** There are hormone-free induction methods which typically come in the form of small thin rods that gradually expand or a small, soft tube with a little inflatable balloon. The principle is that they apply a little bit of pressure on to the cervix to encourage it to open up. For women who have had a previous caesarean section and are having their labour induced, it is usually advised to opt for a hormone-free method like this.

When you have any of these induction methods inserted you can continue to eat, drink and move around as normal. With either method there may be some discomfort once they are in place, but it should not be very painful. This is also a great time to focus on the positioning work we'll discuss in the next chapter.

The purpose of this initial step is to encourage your cervix to open a little so that your waters can be broken in the next step. For some women, this initial step is skipped if their cervix is already softening and opening.

The next step is to make a small hole in the sac of waters around your baby, called artificial rupture of membranes, often abbreviated to ARM. The purpose of this is to allow your waters to start draining and your baby's head to press on to your cervix, encouraging contractions to start. The aim is that this starts contractions in the same way that we discussed in Chapter 8 when your waters break spontaneously. Your body is then given time to see if this is enough to encourage your natural oxytocin to ramp up and contractions to start building. During this time, keeping active and fuelling with food and drink is important, but you can also help your body's natural oxytocin by setting up the positive birth environment you planned in Chapter 5. The process of an induction may take place on a ward where you may or may not have your own room. Even if you don't have your own room, you can still make your bed space feel more comforting and relaxing – you'd also be surprised by the amount of women who make lifelong friends on the maternity wards!

If, after a period of time, your contractions have not yet become regular and powerful, you may be recommended to have a drip of an oxytocin medication. You would be given a very small amount to start with and gradually given a little more until your contractions are coming more regularly. Some women have this oxytocin drip running until their baby is born, while for others it may be turned down or even off as everyone responds differently to oxytocin.

There is a chance that an induction may not be successful, and you then have two potential routes to choose from: either a caesarean section or resting and restarting the induction process. As we have already spoken about, any medical intervention has a balance between risk and benefit, and this balance will look different for all of us and our individual needs and wishes.

I mentioned above that I would talk about some of the pros and cons for induction. This aims to prepare, not scare, you. I want to be totally transparent with you and make sure nothing crops up that you weren't aware of. After reading this I would recommend dipping into some affirmation work like my example on page 16 if you feel any sense of anxiety over induction of labour.

Pros of induction:

- May reduce the risk of a mum or baby becoming unwell if pregnancy continues or birth is left to take place at a later date (some of this is outlined above in the reasons induction may be offered).
- You have an established window of a few days when you know your baby will be born.

Cons of induction:

- You will likely be in hospital a little longer.
- You may be advised to birth in a different setting than you planned, such as a labour ward over home or a birth centre. But remember that you can create the same positive birth bubble in any setting (see Chapter 5).
- The main consideration around using prostaglandins and a synthetic oxytocin drip is that they could cause

too many contractions, which is called hyperstimulation. This is something your midwife will be keeping a close eye out for and there is a medication that can be given to calm this down if it does happen. Pessaries can also be removed and the drip can be switched off.

- May increase your chance of other interventions such as instrumental vaginal birth (see page 135) and complications such as bleeding after birth. There is also evidence to suggest that induction may increase the chance of caesarean section birth:
  - o At 39 weeks 1 in 5 women with spontaneous labour had a caesarean compared to 1 in 3 who were induced.
  - o At 40 weeks 1 in 5 women with spontaneous labour had a caesarean compared to 1 in 3 who were induced.
  - o At 41 weeks 1 in 4 women with spontaneous labour had a caesarean compared to 2 in 5 who were induced.

I hope this highlights how there are potential advantages and disadvantages to induction. As always, it's key to think through your options carefully, speak openly with your midwife and obstetrician, and utilise your decision-making tools from Chapter 6 to support you.

Below are some words of advice from obstetric registrar Laura Kelsey around induction of labour. I hope it helps you to hear that obstetricians are very much on your side. They want you to have a positive experience and to keep you and your baby safe throughout. Their job is to make sure you are aware of the risks and the benefits so you can make informed choices about your care.

Induction of labour is recommended and offered to many people during the course of their pregnancy. It is important that when induction is recommended each individual circumstance is respected. A clear explanation to you about why induction of labour is being recommended, taking into consideration personal risk factors, should be given in a way that you can understand – whether that is presented numerically or with images. There are many circumstances where induction of labour may be offered and, as with many decisions in pregnancy, I recommend you use the BRAIN acronym (see page 98) to support your decision-making.

It is important at each stage of the induction of labour that you are well-informed and empowered to make decisions that are appropriate for you.

If you choose to agree to induction of labour, clinicians can still support you with the things that are important to you. This may include your birth environment (lighting, music), positions in labour and choices at delivery (immediate skin-to-skin, delayed cord clamping and the golden hour, for example). Induction of labour may make up a part of your pregnancy journey, but approaching it well-informed can lead to an empowered, positive birth.

Your obstetrician, like Laura, is there to help you navigate your choices and support you to make an individual care plan. I feel that sometimes obstetricians get a bit of a hard time – the nature of their role means that things often aren't totally smooth-sailing and they may be sharing information you would rather not hear, but if it impacts you and your baby it is important they do tell you. Having a positive relationship with your team, including your obstetrician, will really help you to feel calm and confident in labour. To achieve this and help them be on the same page as you, I would encourage you to be open and talk about what is important to you, vocalise any worries you may have and ask any questions that are troubling you. This can be done verbally, with the support of your birth partner or written on your birth plan, but it will allow your team to meet you where your thoughts are at and answer any of your questions.

IF YOU DECIDE NOT TO HAVE AN INDUCTION

Should you choose to not accept an induction after discussing the advantages and disadvantages for you and your baby, you should next discuss alternatives with your obstetrician and midwife. Alternatives may be an induction at a different time, a planned caesarean section birth or to continue to await spontaneous labour with the option of additional monitoring, such as CTG and ultrasound scanning. It is always important to remember, however, that the CTG and scans do only give a snapshot of your baby at that current situation, and they cannot reliably predict future complications.

'I am able to encourage myself no matter the circumstances I find myself in.'

HOW TO HAVE A POSITIVE INDUCTION OF LABOUR EXPERIENCE

If you decide to have an induction of labour, the first crucial step in ensuring this is a positive experience is to ensure you truly understand why it has been offered to you and that you have had the opportunity to make an informed decision about whether it is the right thing for you and your baby. If you don't feel you have done this at any point, please pause and take some time to ask questions so you have all the information you need. The BRAIN tool from Chapter 6 again comes in very handy here. Remember, this is all your choice.

As you've seen from the various steps in an induction process, it can be a bit lengthy and tiring. Having knowledge of what each step is trying to achieve and being patient is important. Induction is mimicking the process of spontaneous labour – you will remember from Chapter 8 that this is detailed work for your body that can't be rushed, so grant your body the compassion of recognising that it takes time. Ensure you utilise all of the tools and techniques we have discussed in this book – from your mindset prep to your physical prep, breathwork, birthing positions and birthing environment – for each stage of induction as you would for each stage of your labour. Your induction space is yours, so create your birth bubble environment within that. This will support your shy oxytocin hormone (see Chapter 2 for a refresh on the power of oxytocin) to come to the induction party and will, in turn, encourage contractions to start.

I would encourage you to use a birthing ball, do some stretches, walking, squats and lunges regularly throughout your induction of labour as your baby's position can be influenced by how well your body responds to the induction methods. We'll also discuss optimising your baby's position and positions for a better labour and birth, such as 'upright, forwards, open and mobile' and rebozo, in the next chapter, which are super valuable to you during an induction when there can be a temptation to spend prolonged periods of time lying down in a hospital bed.

Keeping occupied and having some distraction techniques can be really helpful if induction takes a few days, so bring some entertainment into the hospital such as music, podcasts or books. Use it as a time to listen to or read positive birth stories (see page 26) and affirmations, and keep snacking and hydrating. Remember, your uterus is a muscle that requires energy to work, just as your car needs petrol or diesel to enable you to drive it.

I found my induction process so smooth. I still felt really in control of my body and, as the contractions grew, I found that breathing techniques helped me to refocus. Out of nowhere, everything intensified, and he was on his way with the aid of a trusty TENS machine and some gas and air. In no time he was in my arms! I actually found this time around really healing mentally from my previous birth and would happily have the same experience again.

Hannah

As a midwife, I have supported many, many women having an induction of labour and the majority of these have a great birth experience. Induction of labour, used appropriately, can be an incredible tool for keeping mums and babies safe, and as a healthcare professional I am so glad we have it available when it is needed. It's so helpful to recognise that there are tools and techniques you can use to aid the process.

PAUSE FOR THOUGHT

Below are some questions to help you plan what a positive induction may look like for you.

- What is the method used at your local hospital? Ask your midwife if you aren't sure and make sure you understand the technique.
- What physical birth preparation techniques do you plan to try (and when) in pregnancy? Refer back to Chapter 4 for ideas on this.
- What will you do in the initial stages of induction to help your body and baby move smoothly through the

process and embrace the little nudge that induction gives you into labour? Consider affirmations and stories from Chapter 1, breathing techniques from Chapter 3 and creating a positive birth environment from Chapter 5.

• What positive affirmation can you create to address a worry of yours over induction of labour? Refer back to Chapter 1 for guidance on how to make your own affirmation that resonates with you on a deeper level.

I hope having some real information about induction helps you shape what this could look like for you.

Next, we're going to look at ways you can move your body to help make your journey through each stage of labour smoother and more comfortable.

REMEMBER:

• You can ask as many questions as you need to when deciding about induction of labour, so take your time and never feel pressurised or rushed into this.

• The risks and benefits to you and your baby will be completely individual so be empowered to make your own decision in conjunction with your medical team.

• You have the right to accept or to decline an induction of labour. Use your BRAIN tool to help you make an informed choice.

12

POSITIONS FOR
A BETTER LABOUR
AND BIRTH

Welcome to one of my favourite chapters and topics. Why? Because what we cover in this chapter – your mobility and the positions you move into during labour and birth – can really influence your labour in a great way. They can lead to a more straightforward journey for your baby through your pelvis and fewer complications. Throughout this chapter, we'll look at why your position is so influential and what the best positions are for birthing your baby.

There is a position for birth that tends to feature in the media, where a woman lies flat on a bed with or without her legs up in stirrups. Sure, this position has its place in some circumstances, but it should be far from your go-to position. You will recall from Chapter 4 the value of optimising your baby's position in pregnancy and how this can reduce birth complications. In an ideal scenario, at the start of labour, your baby is already in an optimal position, and you can then use some of the positions I recommend in this chapter to maintain this and create more space in your pelvis. It is also reassuring to know that, even if your baby is in a back-to-back 'OP' position (see page 62), labour is a great time to change this due to the added power of contractions which can aid your baby's ability to turn.

UPRIGHT, FORWARDS, OPEN AND MOBILE (UFOM) POSITIONS

During labour, you want to adopt positions that allow gravity to work with you and your baby, to improve the descent of your baby through your pelvis and will allow your baby's head to put pressure on your cervix to help it to dilate.

Women often find that certain positions and moving around in between different positions makes contractions easier and more manageable. Being mobile and upright in labour also takes the weight of your bump off the large blood vessels that run down the middle of your abdomen underneath your uterus, and this helps blood to better circulate to your baby and the rest of your body so that you both receive more oxygen.

Now let's look at what positions will really help you. I'll use the acronym UFOM to help you remember:

- **U**pright: Remember, gravity is your friend for helping move your baby downwards during labour. Upright positions such as standing or sitting upright, using a birthing ball or doing some squats and/or lunges will help with this.
- **F**orwards: This is important to encourage your baby into an optimal position for birth as we discussed in Chapter 4. The more forwards your position, the more your baby's back will rotate forwards, which means they are descending through the birth canal with the narrowest diameter of their head, supporting your labour to progress quicker and with fewer complications. Forwards positions also take weight off your tailbone, helping it to move up and out of the way during your baby's descent, and therefore increasing the diameter of

your pelvic outlet that your baby is trying to navigate through. Think of using your upright positions with a forwards lean supported by a chair, bed or your birth partner; all-fours positions are also great for this.

- **O**pen: You want to help make as much space in your pelvis as possible, so your baby has maximum room to move through to be born. A birthing ball or peanut ball are useful for supporting you in open positions (see page 63). Squats and lunges also enable your pelvis to open in different directions, so allow your body to be intuitive. If you find there is a position you are instinctively using, go with it as it is your baby signalling to you the posture they need to help them on their descent. If you do need to lie down, then opt for your left side with your top leg elevated with a peanut ball. A fantastic open pelvis position is to be on all fours with your hands on the floor or supported on a birthing ball or the bed with your knees turned inwards and your ankles turned outwards. This is the reverse to the position you may have seen on TV or in films where ankles are closed and knees are turned out wide. When your knees are close together and your feet and ankles wide, your pelvic diameter opens and helps your tailbone move out of the way, so your baby has a much easier route out.

- **M**obile: Staying mobile and active are also key, so think of moving in and out of the UFO positions regularly. Do some lunges, bounce on a birthing ball, rock, sway and walk to encourage your baby's head to contact the cervix. This, in turn, stimulates more prostaglandins (hormones that help your cervix to soften and open) to be released and signals to your brain to release more oxytocin to help your uterus to contract and labour to progress (see page 75). So don't be afraid to change up your positions, move around and experiment with what feels right to you.

For women with an epidural, adopting some of these positions may be more challenging due to reduced mobility. But there is still lots you can do. Using the peanut ball described above, you can lie on your side with the ball between your legs, or adapt the bed into an upright chair with the bottom of the bed dropped down like a big throne so that you can maintain an upright and open position, even on a bed.

If your baby is having continuous monitoring in labour, you will have some probes attached to your stomach to allow your team to keep a closer eye on baby's heart rate. Please know that this does not mean you must lie on your back on the bed. UFOM positions are for you regardless of what monitoring you are having during labour or what pain relief options you may choose, so I would encourage you to have a chat with your midwife so they can support you to achieve this.

> *I feel my birth experience was so positive, which I feel is due to researching and being educated about UFOM birth positions.*
>
> Annabel

Ideally, start to adopt and practise moving in these UFOM positions in your third trimester and especially from round 36 weeks. This is a great way to help prepare your body for labour and birth, as well as encouraging your baby into that important optimal position. Swap out lounging back on the sofa for left-hand side-lying or, even better, bouncing on your birthing ball and trying some nice forwards yoga poses.

Not sure what these positions look like? Scan the QR code on page 6.

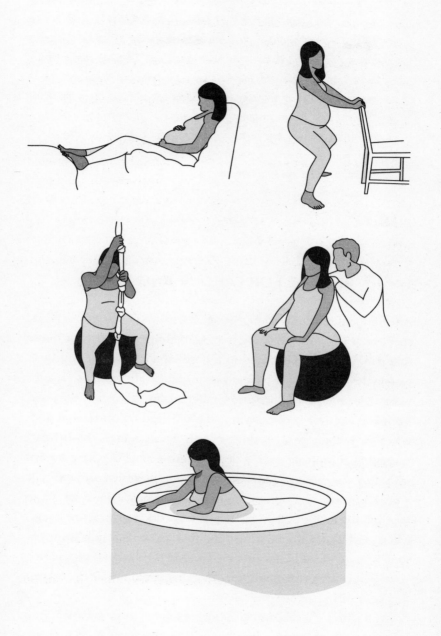

> *In preparing for labour and birth, I learned about UFOM positions and knew I wanted to utilise these. From the beginning of labour, I was experiencing all contractions in my lower back, and I had no choice but to stay upright, lean forwards and keep my pelvis open in order to manage the discomfort. When receiving intermittent monitoring in hospital, baby's heart rate began tracking further around my abdomen, and it became clear that baby had been back-to-back and was now turning (in the final hour of labour!) to optimal birth position. This may not have been possible if I'd been lying down, not adopting UFOM positions, and I could have had a very different birth story!*
>
> Maddy

REBOZO FOR LABOUR AND BIRTH

A traditional rebozo is a long (about 70cm) and wide woven fabric sheet or scarf. You will likely have something around your house that can act as a rebozo and in a hospital a simple flat bed sheet can do the job. They are typically beautiful, brightly coloured cloths worn by women in Mexico and Guatemala for all sorts of life tasks, from keeping warm to carrying children, and by traditional midwives for helping women during birth. I will confess that when I trained as a midwife over a decade ago, I wouldn't have known what this was, but as I have become more interested and more of a geek in birth and optimising baby's positions, I have grown to love rebozo techniques. This is not embedded in practice everywhere and it may not be something your midwife is fully aware of so, if you are keen to use rebozo, I would recommend purchasing your own cloth (or finding something that could mimic it) and getting your birth partner practising.

You can use a rebozo cloth during labour to support you into UFOM positions and to stay in positions like a squat, so they are more effective during labour, allowing you to conserve some valuable energy (and helping out your birth partner's back too). It works well wrapped around your back with a birth partner holding the ends of the rebozo fabric in front of you – this can help take some of the weight off so you can hold a squat for a longer period of time. Another way that a rebozo will be effective is to tie the two ends together in a big, firm knot, then throw the knot over the top of the door and close the door so the rebozo is secured, with a loop on your side. You can then hang off and pull on the rebozo for support and again hold great positions like squats or lunges for longer and with ease.

For many women, just using the rebozo cloth for support in labour is enough. I recall grabbing a wooden beam in our living room in labour and, in hindsight, a rebozo would have been a more comfortable option. But rebozo can also be used to help optimise baby's positions in labour. This is done in a sifting or jiggling motion where you lean over into a hands and knees position and the rebozo is positioned around your stomach. Your birthing partner stands behind you, holding the ends of the rebozo, and jiggles your stomach in a back-and-forth motion. Studies have shown this technique used in labour helps improve the positioning of a baby and has positive physical and physiological benefits.

Another great use for rebozo is to play tug of war with it during the pushing stage of labour. Your birthing partner holds two ends, and you hold the middle of the fabric, and the resistance helps to direct your pushing efforts downwards to help move your baby out. This technique is really helpful for women pushing with an epidural as it can often be more challenging to push as effectively when you have reduced sensation and numbness in this area.

Scan the QR code on page 6 for some videos to help you learn these rebozo techniques.

'Perfectionism is a lie. I give myself permission to start messy and for my birth to unfold in the perfect way for me.'

Moving around and changing positions in labour instinctively around every 20 minutes can be a helpful form of pain relief and allows many women to feel much more comfortable.

In the next chapter we will talk through the pain relief options available to you.

REMEMBER:

- UFOM positions are key to optimising your body and your baby's ability to labour.
- Your birthing partner is great for helping you try different positions during labour, so practise these positions with them and allow them to suggest different ones for you to try during labour.
- No matter what monitoring or pain relief options you opt for during labour, speak with your team to explore UFOM positions that you can achieve in your situation.

13

PAIN REMEDIES AND COMFORT MEASURES

You have many different pain relief methods available to you during labour, and it is a good idea to have an overview of all the options as labour can be unpredictable and you may therefore decide at the time that you wish to try something that wasn't in your original plan. There are also lots of non-medication-based, self-help measures that can really improve your comfort in labour. We will discuss each of these, how they work and their pros and cons throughout this chapter so you are fully informed and know exactly what you can call upon to help you.

I want to reassure you that there will be a comfort measure or pain relief option that will suit you in labour, but it won't necessarily be the same as what your friend, sister or mum used. I encourage you to embrace finding out about all the choices out there and, as always with birth, avoid any sense of comparison and grant yourself the grace to find your own path in birth. A birth without pain relief is not a better or more valid birth than one with – it is your birth and utilising some, or even all, of the methods we will talk through in this chapter will support you to make sure you remain your birth boss and can reflect on your experience in a positive light.

Ultimately, there is no right or wrong pain relief choice.

You can also change your mind or preferences about pain relief at any time and what you may write on your birth preferences now is not set in stone – it can be adapted depending on your situation and feelings at the time.

I trust my instincts and intuition during labour. I am capable of giving birth without fear or anxiety. I am grateful for my body's ability to birth my baby. The pain of labour is temporary, but the joy of holding my baby will last a lifetime.

Kathryn Elizabeth, *My Mountains and Me*

NON-MEDICATION-BASED PAIN RELIEF MEASURES

Often, a sensible approach when navigating pain relief options in labour is to start with lower-level, non-medical measures and move your way through the options as necessary as your labour progresses. Based on this, I have laid these out in the rough order that many women wish to follow in birth.

Education

Just by reading and engaging in this book, having our community group on hand (see page 6 for the QR code) and understanding the processes and your body, you will feel more in control making any pain or discomfort feel less anxiety-provoking as you understand, for example, exactly what a contraction is and can utilise the positive, physiological pain cycle we discussed back in Chapter 1 (see page 23).

Breathing techniques

Use the breathing and relaxation techniques your learned in Chapter 3 as these are your key to keeping calm and drawing focus away from any pain as your contractions rise, peak and fall and you breathe the sensations away.

Positive thoughts and language

Language can be powerful. Try to speak about your birth journey in a positive way, listen to positive birth stories and use positive affirmations because, as you know from Chapter 1, your mind really influences how your body feels too. (Also scan the QR code on page 6 to access some positive birth stories. I know how helpful I found reading these when I was preparing for my own birth.)

Positions

The UFOM and rebozo positions we looked at in Chapter 12 are not only beneficial for supporting your labour to progress well, but they can also be useful in relieving discomfort. (See pages 182 and 186 for a reminder.)

Massage

Massage, especially on your lower back, can be a very effective pain relief measure and is a great way for your birth partner to get involved and help support you.

There are different massage techniques you can use for labour. Some women love the use of massage and touch in their labour, while others don't want to be touched at all – you may know already which personality type you are most likely to be. In my own labour I wanted my husband close and to hold his hand, but other than that I didn't want to be touched. Some women find light stroking called effleurage comforting during labour. This involves your birth partner using a flat hand to lightly stroke your arms, back, shoulders and legs.

It can also be done with the tips of fingers over the abdomen in a feathering method. Your birth partner could provide a shoulder massage, where they sit behind you with their hands on your shoulders and use their hand to stroke downwards from your shoulders in a rhythmic motion to your elbows, using a firm pressure that feels comfortable to you. This is a great technique for helping you to relax and reduce stress and tension, and is great for practising during pregnancy. I also remember getting my husband to give me a shoulder massage a few weeks into breastfeeding postnatally.

Labour can, for some, be felt in the lower back, so the counter-pressure of massage over the lower back can provide great relief with contractions. A flat, firm hand pressure on the lower spine with a contraction can feel great. Simple foot or hand massages can also be relaxing and a great way of incorporating the essential oils we discussed on page 89. I recommend experimenting with some massage techniques ahead of birth so your birth partner is clear on what you do and do not like. Scan the QR code on page 6 for a video of some massage techniques.

Comb acupressure

Squeezing a comb – one that you would use for combing hair – with the pins into the palm of your hand can be an effective coping technique for birth. This technique works because your brain can only focus on a limited number of sensations at a time. By squeezing the comb during a contraction, it may distract your brain and make any painful sensations from the contraction dim down. There is also an acupressure point called the Lao Gong in the palm of your hand which can be triggered when squeezing a comb to help with any painful sensations you may experience. Choose a comb that fits comfortably in your palm and ideally is made from wood to make sure it is strong enough to withstand your squeezing. There is a comb you can buy specifically designed for labour and birth (see Further Resources, page 311, for details).

Birthing partner support

A supportive birthing partner in labour has been shown to reduce the need for medication-based pain relief and birth intervention. So, if possible, be sure to choose a birthing partner who will be positive and reassuring, and communicate your needs to the birthing team.

Water

Being in water is great for adopting UFOM positions (see page 182) because of the way water enables free movement and takes some of the weight off areas that may be feeling achy or uncomfortable in late pregnancy. Some women may choose to birth in the water itself in a bath or birthing pool, whereas others may use it for labour, but not the actual birth. It is an entirely personal choice and is about what feels most comfortable to you at the time. Birthing pools are usually available in a birthing centre or hospital setting and can be hired for use at home births too. Water doesn't just mean water birth though. In the latent phase of labour, you could use showers and baths to provide relief by getting warm water over your bump and lower back.

Using water doesn't stop you using all forms of medication-based pain relief, but it does limit your options. You can't have an epidural while in the water and, if you have an opioid-based pain relief such as pethidine, you will need to wait for the sleepy effects to wear off before getting into a pool. You can still use Entonox (gas and air) in water.

TENS machine

TENS stands for 'transcutaneous electrical nerve stimulation'. A TENS machine is a small electronic device with sticky pads that you can attach to your back. It sends out little electrical impulses that trigger natural endorphins and block the pain signals from reaching your brain. They can work well in the earlier stages of labour, but cannot be used with water due to the electrical component. You can purchase or hire TENS machines for birth and some hospitals have the option to hire them too, but definitely check this before you are admitted.

MEDICATION-BASED OPTIONS

While some women manage their labour without medication-based options, for many (myself included) some can be helpful, and so we will discuss these now. Remember, there is no right or wrong way to manage contractions in labour – every woman and every labour is unique, so try not to compare to others. It is important to do what you need to meet your baby and have a positive and empowering experience.

Oral tablets

Simple paracetamol is safe to take in pregnancy if you have no other contraindications and can also help to ease discomfort, especially in the earlier stages. Your midwife may also advise dihydrocodeine tablets with paracetamol, which give a slightly stronger pain relief. These tend to be best in the latent or early first stage of labour and can be used at home too.

Pros of oral tablets:

- Start to work fairly quickly: within 30 minutes.
- Can provide relief for 4–6 hours.
- Easy to take if you are happy taking tablets.
- Can go home with these tablets.
- Short-term use shouldn't cause side effects.

- Can be used at any stage of labour.
- Can be given in repeat doses 4–6 hourly.

Cons of oral tablets:

- Requires you to take tablets.
- Dihydrocodeine taken regularly can cause constipation.
- Dihydrocodeine may make you feel drowsy/nauseous.
- Not the strongest forms of pain relief available.

Entonox

Entonox, also known as gas and air, is an inhalation form of pain relief. It contains two different gases mixed together: 50 per cent nitrous oxide and 50 per cent oxygen. You simply take deep breaths in and out of a mouthpiece which supplies the Entonox to you. You will be guided to breathe it in as a contraction starts and then stop using it in between contractions to make it most effective for you. Entonox can make contractions feel more bearable and it is also safe for your baby. Entonox is usually used during the first and second stages of labour and can be used for as long as you need. It can also be used if you find any procedures such as VEs too uncomfortable during labour, so speak with your midwife or obstetrician if you feel you may need to use it for these too.

Pros of Entonox:

- Available in any birth setting and you can use it in conjunction with all other types of pain relief.
- You control it yourself by breathing in as much or as little as you wish.

- Entonox works very quickly, within 15–20 seconds, and the slow, deep breaths required can also aid your breathing techniques.
- Can be used for uncomfortable procedures such as VEs.

Cons of Entonox:

- Only recommended for the first and second stages of labour, not the latent phase.
- Some women find that it makes them feel a bit light-headed, tired or nauseous. But should you experience any side effects that you don't like, the good thing is they wear off quickly.
- It can make your lips and mouth feel dry.
- It is short-lasting so needs to be used with every contraction.

Opioids

Diamorphine or pethidine are the most common opioids used for pain relief in labour. The medication is given via injection into a muscle, usually in your thigh or buttock. These are best used in the latent phase or early first stage of labour and are especially useful for women who are tired and struggling to rest and relax.

Pros of opioids:
- Only take around 20 minutes to work and last for, on average, 2–3 hours.
- They help you to relax and cope better with contractions. They often make you feel sleepy and can facilitate

a little nap, which helps rebuild strength for later in labour.

- Repeat doses can be given.

Cons of opioids:

- Opioid injections will usually be offered with an anti-sickness medication, as one of their side effects is nausea and vomiting.
- There may be some short-term pain at the injection site as it is given with a needle.
- Individual reactions vary with these medications and it is not possible to know how effective it will be for you until you try it. For some, they provide more complete pain relief than others but some women find they cause more nausea, dizziness or disorientation.
- You need to wait for the side effects to wear off before getting into a birthing pool or bath.
- We know that these medicines do cross the placenta and so they are best avoided if your baby is close to being born as it can also make them a little drowsy or delay feeding. Your midwife will be able to advise you on the safe and appropriate timing of opioids during your labour.

Epidural

An epidural is an injection into the lower part of your back to block the nerves carrying pain messages from your uterus, which means you stop feeling pain. A fine tube is inserted into your back close to the nerves that supply your uterus so that local anaesthetic can be administered throughout labour. This epidural procedure is done by an anaesthetic doctor who will take your consent and explain all the potential risks prior to doing your epidural. I have summarised some of these below, but your team will be able to advise of any additional or different risks for you based on your personal circumstance. Continuous monitoring of your baby's heart rate is recommended, as discussed in Chapter 5.

The epidural can be put in during the first stage of labour or at any stage as long as you will get benefit from it before you have your baby. The reason I specify this is because commonly in the transition stage of labour we talked about in Chapter 8 (see page 123) women ask for the epidural just before they push their baby out, and this wouldn't be an appropriate time. You do also need to be able to sit or lie still while the epidural is going in, but your team will support you with this and women manage this really well with guidance.

A misconception of the epidural that I feel it is important to address is that it increases the risk of a caesarean section; it does not. It may, however, increase the length of your second stage of labour because you are unlikely to have as much sensation to feel your contractions and pushing urges, and this increases the chance of an instrumental birth. With an epidural, once your cervix is fully dilated, your midwife will usually advise waiting one hour to naturally bring your baby lower in the birth canal before you start pushing. The aim here is to help reduce the length of time you are pushing for.

Pros of epidurals:

- An epidural is usually the most effective form of pain relief and, for 90 per cent of women, gives complete pain relief.
- It usually stays in place until your placenta is delivered and any perineal suturing has been completed, so you will be comfortable throughout those stages too.
- You will be able to rest and sleep and preserve energy.

Cons of epidurals:

- It takes around 40 minutes to take effect, but this may be longer for some women.
- An epidural is only available on a consultant-led unit.
- Around 1 in 10 women will still require some additional pain relief on top of the epidural, such as pethidine or Entonox.
- Your legs tend to become heavy with an epidural, which means that you may not be able to walk around or mobilise so well in labour. However, you can still adopt supported positions on the bed such as left-side-lying with your top leg elevated by a bed stirrup or peanut ball, or an upright chair sitting position, which most beds can now facilitate (see Chapter 12).
- Some hospitals have a policy around not eating with an epidural and may limit fluids to just water.
- The epidural can drop your blood pressure so you will have a cannula sited and some intravenous fluids given to manage this.
- Due to the numb sensation, you may not be able to feel the need to pass urine or be able to spontaneously void urine, so a catheter may be inserted into your bladder if this is the case.
- An epidural is generally a safe form of pain relief. However, as it is a form of intervention, there are potential side effects and risks such as causing nausea, vomiting or itching, and in around 1 per 100 women a severe headache may occur. There are also some more uncommon complications such as infection or nerve damage.

It's worth looking back at the Scales and **BRAIN** tools in Chapter 6 to help you make an informed decision around pain relief options. Here is an example of the **BRAIN** tool in action around the question *'Should I have an epidural?'*:

- Benefits: Will provide great pain relief and allow sleep and rest during labour.
- Risks: May drop my blood pressure. I will need a cannula and fluids through my vein. It may make me itchy. I may not have control of my bladder while it is working so will need a catheter. It will take about 40 minutes to start working. I won't be able to be as mobile. It may increase my chance of a longer pushing stage of labour and the need for assistance through a ventouse or forceps. For 1 in 8 women, it doesn't provide complete pain relief. Around 1 in 100 women have a headache from the epidural.
- Alternatives: I could try other forms of pain relief first.
- Intuition: What is my gut feeling about having an epidural? For example, 'I think I can carry on for another 60 minutes then reassess my thoughts about it' or 'My labour has been very long so far and I really need some rest. I can ask my midwife to support me into a position with the epidural that allows me to keep helping my baby into a good position for birth.'
- Nothing: I could continue without the use of epidural at this time.

I had a really long early stage labour and was in hospital at 3cm due to needing monitoring. I was given morphine as I was struggling with the pain, but it didn't have much effect. On my next check I was 8cm so was given gas and air and it was AMAZING! It didn't take the pain away, but made it so much easier to manage. I'd struggled to eat and drink enough due to the pain, so when I said I fancied a cup of tea, the midwife very quickly made me one. I had gas and air in one hand and a cup of tea in the other, taking sips between contractions. Once on gas and air, it was all I needed to get to 10cm.

Daisy

PAUSE FOR THOUGHT

What stands out for you from these options? For example, do you have an idea of which you may like to try at each stage? Or perhaps you have some questions specific to your individual circumstance that you wish to ask your midwife or obstetrician?

Now you understand the range of pain relief and comfort measures available to you to explore, it's time to talk about supporting your perineum during birth and helping reduce the chance of tearing.

REMEMBER:

- Practising your positive mindset, breathing techniques, squeezing a comb, massage and UFOM positions are effective, risk-free ways to cope with labour.
- Your choice of pain relief may change depending on how your labour journey goes. Having open-minded flexibility about this is really helpful.
- Different pain relief methods may be better suited at different points in your labour. Your midwife will be there to guide you with this and help advise.

14

SUPPORTING YOUR PERINEUM DURING BIRTH

Perineal and vaginal tearing always features high up in the birth fears list and so it is important we delve into it and bust those worries. It is essential to bear in mind that there are so many factors that may influence perineal tearing during birth and there is no definitive way to prevent it – or else we would all be doing it, right?! However, I am dedicating this whole chapter to helping you understand what exactly different types of tears are, ways you can help to reduce the chance of tears and why they don't need to concern you as much as you might think.

One of the first questions most new mums ask me after their baby is born is *'Did I tear?'* Not only does this tell us it's a concern that most of us have, but that we just don't talk about it enough – and, more importantly, it tells me that women do not necessarily feel when a tear has actually taken place. All the nerve fibres are stretched at the point where a tear may occur, so you don't 'feel' it in the same way you may be imagining. So please don't fear this part of labour or let it take an inch of excitement away from the birth of your little one.

I want this chapter to prepare you, not scare you, but I understand that, for some, this may feel like a difficult topic to read about, so you could skip forwards to Chapter 15 if you wish.

Before we look at the different types of tears, I think it's important to remind you that your vagina was designed for birth, so it can stretch considerably to allow your baby to move through it. Your vagina's capacity to stretch and adapt its shape is something that no other muscle has the same ability to achieve. Your perineum is the area of muscle and skin that sits between your vaginal entrance and anus. The perineum is the area most susceptible to tearing during birth. The relaxation phase of your pelvic floor exercises we discussed in Chapter 4 is important for allowing these muscles to relax and soften. Really being able to let everything go, from your jaw and shoulders, through your abdomen and into your pelvis is important when it comes to birth and helping your muscles to function in a fully relaxed state.

> *Childbirth is an experience in a woman's life that holds the power to transform her forever. Passing through these powerful gates – in her own way – remembering all the generations of women who walk with her . . . She is never alone.*
>
> Suzanne Arms, birth advocate and writer

THE DIFFERENT TYPES OF TEARS

Although the vagina and perineal areas are the most common areas of injury post-birth, other areas can be grazed or torn such as the labia, urethra, clitoris, cervix or anus.

Tears to the perineal area are categorised into four types:

- First-degree: Just involving the skin layer and may not require suturing if it isn't bleeding and is well-aligned. Suturing means repairing a tear with stitches that are dissolvable. Anaesthetic is used so you are comfortable throughout the procedure.

- Second-degree: Involves some of the vaginal and/or perineal muscle layer. Suturing would be advised for this type of tear.
- Third- and fourth-degree: For some women (3–4 per cent) the tear may be deeper and extend into the muscle that controls the anal sphincter. These tears will need to be repaired in an operating theatre by an obstetrician with regional analgesia.

HOW COMMON IS TEARING?

For most women, tears are minor and heal without any issues. Around 85 per cent of women sustain some perineal or vaginal trauma during a vaginal birth. With your first baby this risk is a little higher at 90 per cent. I know these statistics may seem high, but as you read on I will explain how some tears are very small and how you can prepare to help minimise tearing. It is also useful to know how common this is because it helps you realise that, if you do have some degree of tearing post-birth, you are not alone, and it shouldn't be a taboo topic to talk about.

Episiotomies

Sometimes a doctor or midwife may, with your consent, make a small cut to the perineum. This is called an episiotomy. An episiotomy makes the opening of the vagina a bit wider, allowing the baby to come through it more easily. They are not performed routinely and are only done to create extra space away from the anus to try to prevent a tear going into the anal sphincter (third- and fourth-degree tears) or speed up birth if there are concerns over your or your baby's well-being and your baby needs to be born a little quicker. They are also performed with assisted births, as we discussed earlier (see page 137).

How tears are repaired

Your midwife or obstetrician will offer to examine your vagina and anus after you give birth to determine if there is a tear and what type it is. This is recommended following all vaginal births as a tear may not always be visible on the outside. This involves a gentle examination of the tissues with your consent and a finger being placed in your rectum to feel for any injury such as third- or fourth-degree tears. Pain relief is provided for the assessment of tearing post-birth and it will only be performed with your consent.

Any tears or trauma are repaired after birth with your consent using dissolvable sutures and pain relief is provided for this procedure so you will be comfortable. You can continue to have skin-to-skin with your baby during this procedure. Most tears will be repaired in the same room you gave birth to your baby in, except third- or fourth-degree tears which would be repaired in a theatre room instead. If you birth at home, your midwife will recommend using a bed or sofa for a repair. If you were to sustain a third- or fourth-degree tear it would be recommended to transfer into hospital as this cannot be repaired at home and needs to be done by an obstetrician.

HOW TO REDUCE THE RISK OF TEARING

There is some evidence that some measures may help to reduce the risk of or the severity of tears. You may wish to give some of these a go:

- **The position you give birth in:** Being in upright and mobile positions during birth can reduce the risk of tearing (see Chapter 12 for the benefits of UFOM birth positions).

- **Warm compress:** The use of a warm compress, such as gauze or a maternity pad soaked in warm water, held onto your perineum by your midwife during the final stages of birth as your baby's head is crowning has been shown to increase the chance of your perineum being intact and reduce the chance of episiotomy and more severe tearing. This is the simplest thing to do and the 'Warm Pack trial' has shown this technique can halve the rate of severe perineal tears. You can ask your midwife for this and, as long as your birthing position allows, they should be happy to support you. If you birth in a pool, the water provides this for you so there is no need for a warm compress too. I literally see women's faces relax when a warm compress is applied – it is such a soothing sensation in the final stages of birth.

- **Perineal support techniques:** Your midwife can, with your consent, support your perineum by placing a hand on the back part of your vulva and perineum as your baby's head is born. This is something you can ask for and your midwife may routinely offer it to you, but, to cover all bases, you can add this to your birth preference list and discuss it with your team ahead of your birth. This gentle support to your perineum has been shown to decrease the chance of third- or fourth-degree tears. This is not possible when birthing in water, but birthing in water has also been shown to reduce the risk of more severe tearing during birth.

- **Breathing techniques:** At the time of your baby's head crowning, use your downwards breath from Chapter 3 or blow like you are blowing out birthday candles on a cake to allow for a more controlled birth of your baby's head rather than big pushes. Breathing or blowing rather than pushing as your baby's head is born slows the process and allows time for your tissues to stretch rather than one big stretch all at once, and may also reduce the chance of more significant tearing.

- **Perineal massage:** Massaging the areas of your vagina and perineum that are most susceptible to injury during birth to gently encourage some stretch and to improve the elasticity of the tissues has been shown to reduce the length of the pushing stage of labour, and reduce the risk of tearing and episiotomy, including reduced third- and fourth-degree tears. It has also been shown to improve wound healing, perineal comfort and to lower the risk of bowel incontinence postnatally. You can start performing perineal massage from 34 weeks in your pregnancy and it is recommended to do the massage 3–4 times a week, for around 3 or 4 minutes at a time. If you have a vaginal infection such as thrush or active herpes, then it is best to avoid perineal massage.

  If the potential benefits of perineal massage sound good to you, take a look at the box below for an explanation of how to perform it.

- **Pelvic floor exercises:** We discussed how to perform your pelvic floor exercises in Chapter 4 and why they are important for pelvic floor health during pregnancy and the postpartum. But performing them alongside perineal massage has also been shown to increase the chance of having no tearing from 6 per cent to 17 per cent as well as reducing perineal pain post-birth and lowering the chance of experiencing urinary incontinence.

HOW TO PERFORM PERINEAL MASSAGE

The idea is to gently massage and stretch the muscles at the opening of your vagina and the perineal tissues.

1. Sit comfortably with clean hands, a mirror and some lubricant (either natural oils or a water-based lubricant work well).

2. Place your thumbs about 2.5–4cm just inside the back wall of your vagina and press down towards your anus and to the sides. Hold this stretch for 1–2 minutes.

3. Gently move to the lower bit of your vagina for 2–3 minutes, focusing on relaxing your perineum and massaging in a U-shaped movement.

4. You could practise your slow, deep breathing techniques (from Chapter 3) while you do this. It should not be painful, though you may feel a slight stretching sensation as you massage the area.

It may help you to see perineal massage in a video – scan the QR code on page 6. If you are finding the reach over your bump a struggle, you can ask your partner to help you.

I did my research and started perineal massage at 36 weeks, as well as regular pelvic floor exercises. I knew that, despite this, my chances of tearing were still high as a first-time mum. After 40 minutes of pushing there were concerning features on the CTG and we decided the best course of action was a ventouse delivery and episiotomy. I was scared about the episiotomy, but the team reassured me it was the best way to protect my perineum during an instrumental birth. The doctor used local anaesthetic so I didn't feel a thing when she performed the procedure. My baby was born quickly and safely and I didn't even realise the doctor had begun stitching because I was too engrossed in the tiny beautiful human in my arms. For the next few days I found a more comfortable sitting position and kept topped up with simple painkillers. Going for a wee was no different to before and, despite much anticipation, the first poo was absolutely fine! I didn't even need any of the fancy products I had bought. At my ten-day check-up the midwife informed me it had completely healed and, four months down the line, I wouldn't know anything had even come out of there! I wish I hadn't been so worried about tearing or needing an episiotomy. This was a decision I made in the best interests of me and my baby.

Fran

PAUSE FOR THOUGHT

This is your space to pause and reflect on how you feel about this topic after reading the information above, to take down any notes you would like to add into your birth preferences and reminders for when you will start your perineal prep.

If you have stuck with me throughout this chapter, well done, because I know it is a topic that may have made you cross your legs at the start. You should hopefully now feel better prepared for how you can help your perineum and, crucially, to know that tearing is common so, if you do have a tear, it is not a taboo – I had a tear during birth and all is well!

Hopefully you are starting to realise how all the work you have done through the earlier chapters on your physical and psychological preparation is linking into all aspects of your birth journey, including your perineum and ways you can help to reduce damage and improve recovery.

Another key way to prepare is to get your birth partner on board and knowledgeable. Birthing partners are so important and, for this reason, the next chapter is dedicated to them.

REMEMBER:

- Tearing during vaginal birth is common, but there are things you can do to reduce the chance and degree of tearing you may experience.
- The use of a warm compress and slow, controlled breathing will help reduce discomfort at this stage of your birth.
- Your anatomy was designed for this and has incredible stretching abilities and healing potential.

15

HOW TO BE THE ULTIMATE BIRTH PARTNER

Birth partners are so important in labour and birth, but sometimes they can feel like they are a bystander – just waiting by the sides, feeling a little awkward with all the vagina and breast talk going on, unsure of their role and what they can do to help. So, I am writing this chapter directly to all you birth-partners-to-be to empower and educate you so you can really boss your important role, enjoy the experience and create a powerful bond with your partner and baby throughout your journey.

This chapter can also be read by any mums-to-be and I would also really welcome and encourage birth partners to read more than just this chapter. Ideally, you would read this book cover to cover, so you too understand the processes of birth and what to expect.

BIRTH PARTNERS ARE POWERFUL

As a birth partner, I recommend being open to immersing yourself in birth and parenthood education. Everyone is going to benefit from you being a knowledgeable and involved birth partner. So,

say this aloud with me, 'evidence shows that a supportive birth partner increases the likelihood of a spontaneous vaginal birth, shortens
the length of labour, reduces the chance of intervention (including
caesarean sections) and improves maternal experience'. That supportive person is YOU.

You are not an awkward bystander;
you are fundamental in this birth and you are
on a journey too.

Now, as we talk about the role of a birth partner, it is important
you feel confident and on board with this role and that we can be
honest in recognising it is not for everyone – and that is absolutely
OK. Having open and honest conversations about who is best
placed to fulfil this role or if perhaps a second birth partner is a
good idea is important. Most hospitals and birthing units in the
UK allow two birthing partners to be present. You can, of course,
ask your midwife how many are routinely accepted at your local
unit to be sure. A benefit to home birth is that you can have as
many birth partners with you as you like and there are no visiting
time restrictions as there would be in a hospital. However, if your
partner labours in hospital, the birthing partner can be present for
the duration of the birth and isn't required to stick to visiting times
that may otherwise apply. These are logistics that are useful to ask
about beforehand so you don't have any surprises at the time and
can plan ahead.

*Antenatal prep is so important. Take the time to really understand the
preferences of the person you're supporting in various circumstances. It
was helpful understanding exactly what Ali would opt for as things*

unfolded – while she had an ideal scenario in mind, the reality deviated somewhat. Chances are there will come a point when they need your help to articulate these preferences for them. I found it helpful to understand what was really important to her versus what were nice-to-haves.

Jack

WAYS TO PROVIDE PRACTICAL SUPPORT

Let's start with some of the practical ways in which you can provide support as a birth partner.

Encouraging eating and drinking

Remember, the uterus is a muscle and, just like any other muscle, it needs fuel to contract. We aren't talking full-blown meals in labour, but encouraging your partner to nibble on cereal bars, sweets and foods that will give some energy is perfect. Hydration is also important in labour as mums often forget to drink, so having a sports bottle handy that you can easily pass across in between contractions for little sips is a great idea.

Taking charge of the birthing environment

If you haven't read Chapter 5, please do so now because this is one of your key roles. The birth environment is crucial to allowing labour to progress and improves the chance of birth being a positive experience. Communicate together ahead of time about what this is going to look like so you know exactly what you need to do and can take charge of it. If you need assistance, you can ask your midwife too. Things to think about include: sorting and maintaining the agreed lighting, music and scents.

Supporting different positions

You can be a great support in allowing your partner to move into more comfortable labour positions. The rebozo techniques will help you with this (see Chapter 12 on positions for labour and birth). I recommend changing positions regularly during labour and birth, especially during the pushing stage if things are taking longer than expected (every 20 minutes or so). Do encourage movement – a trip to the bathroom, positional adjustments or a walk around the room will all help baby to navigate through the pelvis.

Keeping her cool

A handheld fan and cold flannel should also be within reach of any birth partner. Labour is hot, often sweaty, work and helping mum-to-be feel comfortable and cool makes a big difference.

Using massage

Massage can be a great comfort and form of pain relief, and has actually been shown to reduce the need for pharmacological pain relief during labour. The lower back area is usually the most beneficial area to provide massage in labour and can be done with your hand or a handheld massage tool. If aromatherapy is on your list, then massaging in the oils is a lovely option. Have a peek back at Chapter 13, if you haven't read it already, where there is more information on massage techniques you can use.

Practising your hair and beauty skills

OK, you don't need to be ready to glam up the stars here, but wispy bits of hair can be really infuriating. Having a hairband to hand or being able to do a basic ponytail will get you some brownie points, as will passing the lip balm when your partner's lips start to look dry (hospital air and Entonox are notorious for drying out lips).

Announcing baby's sex

If you don't know what sex you are expecting, it can be really lovely for birth partners to be the first to announce this. If this is something you would like to do, just let your midwife know ahead of time so they don't accidentally say. If gender is not something you wish to focus on, then of course you can skip this.

Cutting the cord

Birthing partners can also cut the umbilical cord once the baby is born if they wish. If this makes you feel squeamish, remain open-minded and decide at the time. My husband was certain this was not a job for him, but when it came to the birth of our son, there was no stopping him. Often birth partners do change their mind about this when caught up in the oxytocin, love bubble of a new baby.

Skin-to-skin

We hear lots about mums having skin-to-skin (and we will cover this in Chapter 17), but if you are also the baby's parent, skin-to-skin for birth partners can be a lovely bonding time too. Should there be a need to separate mum and baby at birth, please do not be afraid of skin-to-skin as it is a great way to support your baby to regulate their heartbeat and maintain their temperature. Remember, babies can also hear in the womb from around 18 weeks of pregnancy, so your voice may be familiar and soothing to them in the new outside world. You might want to try calmly talking or even singing to them when they are born to help comfort them.

HAVE THE CAMERA READY

Do you want photographs or videos during labour or when baby is born? This comes down to personal choice, but your team will be happy to support this. They may wish to not be included in any imagery or videos, so talk this through beforehand.

When your partner goes into labour, what she needs most from you is for you to do the 'thinking' while she focuses on the 'birthing'. Make sure you know the birth plan, where everything is in the hospital bags and what her pain relief preferences are. When she's in the thick of it, she'll be relying on you to advocate for her, but don't worry, the midwives will be on hand and are really good at supporting you too. Tell her she's doing a great job, get her lots of water if she needs it, and be on hand to help her in her labour positions and with her breathwork. And, finally, if she says she needs gas and air, for the love of God, give it to her!

Daniel

WAYS TO PROVIDE PSYCHOLOGICAL SUPPORT

As a birth partner, you can also provide some much-needed psychological support.

Touch and encouragement

Hand-holding, words of support and encouragement or even using some positive birth affirmations (you will find some of these dotted through the chapters of this book, but of course you can find your own too) will also help mum-to-be to stay positive and remind her how strong and capable she is. Have some affirmations you both like to hand and you can read these to your partner during birth to keep her positive mindset on track.

Advocate

As a birth partner, you have a crucial role as an advocate, ensuring your partner's wishes are known and catered for by the team. You can also use the BRAIN tool discussed in Chapter 6 to ask questions to ensure you all fully understand the pregnancy and birth options throughout. Below is an example of the BRAIN tool in action for a birth partner.

USING THE BRAIN TOOL AS A BIRTH PARTNER

'Should I try offering massage?'

- Benefits: It may help provide relief from contractions and aid relaxation.
- Risks: My technique might not be spot on. It may not ease the contractions like I hope.
- Alternatives: I could try other forms of support like helping with breath control and using affirmations. I could also use a massage tool to provide massage instead of my hands, which may be easier.
- Intuition: What is my gut feeling about offering massage? How did it work when we practised it ahead of birth?
- Nothing: I could continue supporting without offering massage.

With all of this to do, you will have no time to be an awkward bystander – you have a super important and empowering role here.

PROTECTING BIRTH PARTNERS

The old saying that you can't care for someone else if you don't care for yourself is really relevant to you as a birth partner. You need to make sure you are eating and drinking too and have personal care items like toothpaste, deodorant and clean clothing in case you are in hospital for a while (see page 105 for my top recommendations on what to pack).

Another important reason for you to be educated and informed ahead of your partner's birth is to help reduce their chance of experiencing birth trauma. Birth trauma has been traditionally associated with the birthing woman, but the reality is there are many people impacted by birth trauma who are not the ones giving birth. Birth partners can be vulnerable in the birth setting, especially if they have gone into it without preparation. In the set-up of a birth room, the birth partner has a bird's eye view of everything that is happening – they see all the facial expressions and hear all the conversations. This can be overwhelming and scary if there is a complication, which can leave them at an increased risk of birth trauma or post-traumatic stress disorder (PTSD). There are details for the Birth Trauma Association in the Further Resources, page 113, should you or your partner be impacted by trauma during birth.

YOUR BIRTH PARTNER ACTION PLAN

We must recognise that every woman's needs are unique, and this is why I recommend you make a short checklist after communicating together about what your birth partner role should be. This mini checklist allows you to be clear on what your partner feels she needs from you and what you feel able to give and facilitate. For example, some women love to be touched or spoken to during contractions, while others want to be left alone and undisturbed – neither is wrong, it is just the way we differ in personality.

Top tip: Have a copy of this in your pocket or on your phone during birth – it is like your birth to-do list.

As a birth partner, being well-informed and educated about birth allows you to not just boss being a birth partner, but to enjoy the experience yourself too.

REMEMBER:

- The role of a birth partner is an active, involved and supportive one.
- Communication is key: know exactly what the person you are supporting wants so you feel confident in your role.
- You are important too. Make sure you have things with you to meet your basic needs, such as food and drink, a phone charger and a change of clothes.

16

IT IS TIME TO CREATE YOUR BIRTH PREFERENCES

We have discussed lots of information throughout Parts 1 and 2 and hopefully you are starting to form your own ideas and visions about what you would like for your birth. You have jotted down key information and your thoughts from the reflective pauses. Now it is time to bring this all together into one place so that you, your birth partner, midwife and obstetrician are also all aware of your wishes.

PREFERENCES OVER PLANS

You have likely heard the term 'birth plan', but I prefer to use the term 'preferences'. As you are now aware (but hopefully not now fearful of the fact), sometimes things do not go to plan, and twists and turns can crop up along the way. With this in mind, you can see why having a set 'plan' when it comes to birth isn't so helpful. Instead, looking at what you would like to happen in each scenario and having your decision-making tools and coping techniques to hand is a more useful and realistic way to prepare for a positive birthing experience.

I am naturally organised and love planning ahead. The spontaneity and lack of control of birth didn't suit my personality and made me quite anxious. But I learned that I had choices and was able to put together my birthing plan. It gave me the feeling of being in control and, as strange as it sounds, allowed me to enjoy giving birth.

Jessica

HOW TO WRITE YOUR BIRTH PREFERENCES

Creating a birth preferences list is helpful in allowing clear communication between you and your care provider, and for helping you to navigate your options and choices. It's good to have thought about and written down your birth preferences by 36 weeks.

As you complete your preferences and consider what is most important to protecting a calm and positive birthing space for you, I encourage you to also consider how you will replicate this across a variety of birth settings, as we talked about in Chapter 5. Get your birth partner involved with creating your preferences so they understand how they can help facilitate the birth you would like and feel confident in their roles and responsibilities.

It can be easier to use a structure to create your birth preferences, so I have provided a planner for you on pages 226–7. This will allow you to easily communicate what is important to you during your birth so your birth partner and medical team can help facilitate your preferences and support you to have the positive and empowered birthing experience you totally deserve. Some women prefer to write their birth plan and pass it to their midwife, whereas others prefer to verbalise their wishes at the time or even a combination, but either way having it written down allows you and your birth partner to be clear on your wishes and to consider the twists and turns.

Where I see birth preferences work best is when they have flexibility and consideration for all avenues that birth can follow. Where they don't seem to work so well is when there is a very strict, regimented plan and blanket rules around certain options, which can be challenging when there is a deviation. Ultimately, we don't know what may suit us best until we are there going through it, so having an open mind is helpful.

Sometimes, when you write down what you would like from your birth it can feel like you are asking for something out of the ordinary or asking too much. But, remember, this is one special day in your life and you will be able to create powerful memories by putting your stamp on it. Your birth is yours and your midwife and team are there to support you, to ensure it is an experience you can treasure and so you can step into parenthood adjusting your superwoman cape feeling strong, capable and empowered by your journey.

The detail is important and often the most powerful influences are the small things: the words of a certain song that resonate, the lip balm for dry lips, the cool flannel on a sweaty brow. These may seem like unimportant things, but they make the world of difference in allowing you to be calm, relaxed and comfortable as your body and baby whirl through the magical dance of labour together. Know that from these two parts of the book and all the little exercises you have done, your toolbox for managing your labour and birth is piled high and you have set yourself up in a great place to do this.

BIRTH PREFERENCE PLANNER

My name: _____

Birth partner: _____

I wish to birth at:
_____

We're expecting:
a girl ☐
a boy ☐
don't know ☐

My preferred positions for labour and birth:
_____
_____
_____
_____

My birth environment:
Dim lighting ☐
Music ☐
Aromatherapy ☐

Battery candles ☐
Skin-to-skin ☐
Delayed cord clamping ☐

If my birth takes place in theatre, I wish the above environment to be replicated as far as possible ☐

If dim lighting isn't possible, I have an eye mask ☐

My preferred analgesia options:
_____
_____
_____
_____

Cord to be cut by:
_____

3rd stage of labour:
Active ☐
Physiological ☐

I would like to:
Breastfeed ☐
Formula feed ☐
Combination feed ☐

Vitamin K:
Injection ☐
Oral ☐
None ☐

Additional notes / wishes:

_____

_____

_____

_____

_____

_____

_____

_____

_____

_____

_____

_____

_____

_____

_____

_____

_____

BIRTH PREFERENCE PLANNER

*'You are stronger than you think and more
capable than you know.'*

You are not on this journey alone; there are hundreds of babies around the world being born at the exact same minute that your baby is born – allow yourself to feel the strength of doing this with other women.

REMEMBER:

- Preferences are important in shaping your positive birth, but have flexibility and be open to adapting if needed.
- Communicate your preferences with your birth partner so they can help facilitate these – my husband was in charge of my birth environment in our son's birth.
- You have so much inner strength and capability, as well as a toolbox packed with tools and techniques to boss your birth, however that may be for you and your baby.

PART 2
REFLECTION

You have completed Part 2! Your birth preparation knowledge is supercharged and you have all the information in these pages to be well-informed ahead of your birth.

We have discussed a lot in this part of the book, and it is detailed and intricate in places, so do not feel you must have all of your plans, preferences and wishes nailed down right now. If you do, that is great, but if you do not, give yourself some time, space and compassion to absorb what we have covered, reflect or even reread elements as you need to. I hope you'll then feel empowered to shape your birth wishes in your own time.

You may find some chapters have brought up questions and you need to speak with your obstetrician or midwife about them and that is fantastic too, so note down these thoughts ready for your next appointment. If you need some time to consider the elements of Part 2 more before moving into Part 3 I recommend scanning the QR code on page 6 and reading some of the birth stories as these may also spark ideas for you.

Before we move into Part 3 and explore the postpartum period, please know that you can do this – you have everything within you to birth your baby by whatever means, and the team of experts around you will guide, advise and support you to boss your birth.

QUIZ

Here is our Part 2 quiz to help you consolidate the knowledge and takeaways we have covered. As before, all the answers are on page 309 for you to check your new knowledge.

1. What are the different stages of labour?
2. What hormone surges during the transition stage?
3. What is the acronym for your labour and birth positions?
4. In what birthing place is an epidural available?
5. What's the name of the two instruments that may be used in an assisted vaginal birth?
6. How common is a caesarean section birth?
7. From how many weeks can you begin perineal massage?
8. When should you complete your birth preferences?

Jot down any key take-homes from Part 2 in the space below:

_____

_____

_____

_____

_____

_____

_____

PART 3
You Did It: Immediately Post-Birth

And just like that, you enter the beautiful whirlwind of parenthood. Commonly the first 12 weeks postpartum is termed the 'fourth trimester' and I love that this period is given its own recognition because it really is a huge time of change, transition and recovery for mums, babies and the whole family unit.

I would honestly need a complete other book to talk about every aspect of the fourth trimester (added to my to-do list: write a second book), but I also don't feel I can provide you with the very best guide to a positive birth without talking about the immediate postpartum period as it is so closely related to your birth experience.

Towards the end of your pregnancy, it's a great idea to think about ways in which you can prepare for these first few weeks to help your transition into motherhood. The reality is, though, that no one can tell you exactly what your postpartum recovery will be like as everyone's journey is so unique. However, there are some things that you can do to ease the pressure, support a smoother transition and manage the challenges of the early postpartum.

The wise words of psychotherapist and bestselling author Anna Mathur resonated with me throughout my postpartum journey, and I want to share these with you too before we embark on this final part of the book:

> We have the idealism of a Mary Poppins-style mother – it is all perfect and unattainable – and at the other end of the spectrum we have the Incredible Hulk, where overwhelm, exhaustion and frustration has built up inside us.

My happiest place in the immediate postpartum was when I found a middle ground between these two characters, recognised perfection doesn't exist in the real-life world and that I needed to communicate and take care of myself to not allow the Hulk to take over. I often visualise myself even now sliding along a line between these two and making sure I can keep some balance somewhere in the middle.

17

THE GOLDEN HOUR AND BONDING WITH YOUR BABY

That moment when your little one is handed to you for the first time is magical. As a midwife, it still gets me every time and there is honestly no way to describe it. As the saying goes, 'not only is a baby born, but so is a mother'. It is easy to rush through this initial period of time together in the blink of an eye, or while on the phone sharing the news, but I encourage you to pause and be intentionally present in this newly-born period.

The immediate hour following your birth is commonly named the 'golden hour' and for good reason. As your baby is born, they are suddenly in a completely different world to the cosy, warm and secure space they have known in your uterus. All the things that have been regulated for them become things they now have to manage for themselves. You have also been waiting a long time to see your little one's face, smell them and hold them in your arms. So, take a pause and enjoy this special moment.

THE GOLDEN HOUR AND BREASTFEEDING

The golden hour is a golden opportunity to bond, initiate and help establish breastfeeding. Having lots of uninterrupted skin-to-skin with your baby in this hour also helps them to experience a gentler transition into the outside world.

There are nine stages you will notice your baby cycle through in their first hour of life if you watch them closely:

1. First cry. When your baby is born they will usually, if there are no complications, let out a loud distinctive cry as their lungs aerate for the first time and they take their first breath.
2. Relaxation. Following their initial cry, with skin-to-skin, your baby then relaxes and you will notice they become much more still and calm.
3. Awakening. After a short relaxation, your baby will begin to open their eyes, blink a little and make small movements with their hands. It is common to notice some suckling movements with their mouth in this stage too.
4. Activity. Following the more gentle and subtle awakening stage, your baby begins larger movements where they may move their whole arms around and lift their head up a little.
5. Rest. This new activity is very stimulating for your baby so they will regularly disperse short periods of movement with longer, restful periods.
6. Crawling. It is not the type of crawling on all fours across the floor, but in skin-to-skin your baby will attempt to navigate to the breast. This may involve a bobbing, sliding or pushing motion.
7. Familiarisation. Once at or near your nipple, your baby will move their tongue to lick at the area, smell, taste and touch with their mouth and hands to familiarise themselves.

8. **Sucking.** After familiarising and navigating your nipple and breast, your baby will attempt to latch and suck at the breast for their first breastfeed if this is how you have chosen to feed your baby.

9. **Sleep.** One-and-a-half to two hours after birth, following a feed, your baby will rest to sleep.

Uninterrupted skin-to-skin during this time helps to increase your oxytocin, the love hormone, which in turn helps promote breast-feeding. To initiate this all-important milk-production mechanism, try to feed your baby in this first hour if possible. Mothers and babies who have immediate skin-to-skin contact have been shown to have higher rates of exclusive breastfeeding, to be more likely to still be breastfeeding at four months and to breastfeed for longer. Of course, not all mothers will be able to have the first hour as uninterrupted skin-to-skin if there is a medical reason why a mum or baby needs care or monitoring, but do not worry – there are still great benefits to skin-to-skin contact at other times too. There is a section in this chapter for you to help navigate any separation (see page 239).

The latest infant feeding survey showed that 81 per cent of mothers initiate breastfeeding, but this falls to 24 per cent of babies being exclusively breastfed at six weeks, and only 1 per cent at six months. The World Health Organization recommends that 'children initiate breastfeeding within the first hour of birth and be exclusively breastfed for the first six months of life – from the age of six months, children should begin eating safe and adequate complementary foods while continuing to breastfeed for up to two years of age or beyond'. The closeness of skin-to-skin between you and your baby in this golden hour allows for both of your instinct-ive behaviours to be triggered and it is exciting to know that a simple step like skin-to-skin in the uninterrupted golden hour can help with breastfeeding success. Allowing your baby to attach to the breast early and achieve self-attachment means they are likely to remember how to breastfeed at future feeds, and this can help prevent breastfeeding problems arising. This closeness and contact support the release of your milk supply hormones too. Skin-to-skin and early breastfeeding in the golden hour has been linked to improve short- and long-term milk supply in mothers, which helps you have a smoother breastfeeding journey without low supply issues cropping up. We will discuss feeding options in Chapter 18. You may already have an idea about how you wish to feed your baby or you may be undecided at the moment – as always, it is your body and your choice.

THE POWER OF THE GOLDEN HOUR FOR MOTHER AND BABY

Skin-to-skin and the golden hour are not only for mothers who wish to breastfeed – the benefits are for your baby's health and well-being too. Skin-to-skin contact supports your baby to regulate their temperature, oxygen saturations, blood sugar control and breathing when they are born, and these are key things that are essential to your baby thriving and remaining well in the early days of newborn life. Remember, it is the first time they have needed to breathe for themselves, and the outside world looks and feels very different to being inside of you.

Skin-to-skin is also a brilliant way to promote the transfer of your good bacteria to your baby's skin, which supports the important development of their microbiome. Babies who are born vaginally benefit from the colonisation of their mother's vaginal microbiome as they pass through the birth canal. Babies born via caesarean section do not receive this so skin-to-skin is an extra beneficial tool to support the microbiome of caesarean-born babies. Emerging research on this topic links gut microbiome to reduced incidence of infections and allergy conditions such as eczema, asthma and allergies in babies. Your arms are the perfect place for your baby to be as they transition to the outside world.

Having time with your new baby to cuddle in skin-to-skin, look at and really take in their brand-new beautifulness in this golden hour doesn't only benefit them, it is great for your health too. Once your baby is born, there is a surge of oxytocin to help contract your uterus and protect you against excessive bleeding. When you have skin-to-skin it helps to boost this oxytocin level and having close contact with your baby during this time helps to trigger bonding between you both. Furthermore, as improved bonding is protect- ive against postnatal depression, skin-to-skin supports your mental as well as your physical health.

During your golden hour, your baby can have delayed cord clamping, which has incredible benefits (see Chapter 8). Routine things such as weighing your baby can all wait until you are ready, so don't feel you need to interrupt your golden hour if all is well and you are enjoying the cuddles. You can still have this time if you have a caesarean section birth – just speak with your midwife so they can support your wishes.

Skin-to-skin is beneficial at any time so enjoy as much of it as you wish. I always used to start my day with our newborn son with a skin-to-skin feed in bed while my husband made my breakfast, and then we would swap and he would have skin-to-skin while I ate my breakfast and grabbed a quick shower. No matter what our night had entailed, this was like a morning reset and set us all up for a calm day.

It is also important to say that while some parents report an overwhelming instantaneous rush of love at the birth of their little one, this feeling can also take time and need some support to feel that love and connection. Be kind and gracious to yourself – all emotions and feelings are valid during this time and every journey to parenthood looks different, so varying responses are expected.

Birth can be quite an overwhelming experience and those feelings of intense love can take a while.

If you are concerned about your ability to bond with your baby, this can be a sign of postnatal depression (PND). We will discuss this in Chapter 19 so you are aware of things to keep an eye out for. It is important to not feel guilty or ashamed about this and to speak with your midwife or health visitor. This is more common than you may realise and there is help and support services available. There are some further resources on page 311 for anyone experiencing bonding or mental health concerns – you are not alone and things can get better with the right help.

WHEN THE GOLDEN HOUR ISN'T IMMEDIATELY POSSIBLE

Sometimes, although uncommon, mums and babies may be separated after birth for a period of time, or a mum may have given birth under a general anaesthetic and the immediate golden hour is not possible. Please try not to worry about this – keeping you and your little one safe and well is the top priority. When you are reunited with your baby, you can start skin-to-skin straight away and have your golden hour then instead. You will still get huge benefits and can continue to have as much skin-to-skin as you wish over the early hours, days and weeks with your baby. The teams caring for you both will be keen to get you back together as soon as possible and they will support bonding opportunities, such as taking lots of pictures and videos of your baby and having a piece of cloth or a small teddy that you can swap so you can smell each other and feel closer.

I've included some tips below from a neonatal mum, Jessica, and neonatal nurse, Carys, to help you navigate any time when you are separated from your baby or when they are in NICU to ensure you feel less worried and are still able to be involved with their care and bond with them.

TOP TIPS FOR SUPPORTING BONDING

Jessica says:

- Don't be afraid to ask questions.
- Get involved when you can. My husband's first ever nappy change was through the incubator arm holes under the kind guidance of a nurse!
- Document milestones and take pictures – for example, when baby comes off oxygen or when the nasal tubes come out, your first cuddle, and so on. It's nice to see how far you have come when the days blur together and to look back on later on.

TOP TIPS FOR REDUCING WORRY

Carys advises:

- When there are no changes to your baby's care plans, it doesn't mean there is no progress. Static is good – it means your baby is growing and getting ready to reach that next milestone.
- Neonatal nursing is sometimes more like an art form than a science because every baby is different; it's not a one-size-fits-all approach. Some babies are slow and steady, while some 'run before they can walk' so can have setbacks. With this in mind, as a professional, it can be really hard to give you a clear idea of your NICU journey, so try not to worry if things feel a bit vague – your baby is in safe hands.

Although the 'golden hour' may not be immediately possible with unwell or preterm babies who require more support at birth, skin-to-skin and a little cuddle for a shorter period of time may still be achievable and is of great benefit to both mum and baby. I worked with a team on a project called 'Delivery Room Cuddles' where we provided skilled care to babies born under 32 weeks in skin-to-skin with their mothers. The outcomes showed no poor effects on babies and even improvements to their stabilisation when their immediate post-birth care was provided in close skin-to-skin contact with their mum. The power of a mummy (and daddy) cuddle is phenomenal. If Mum is unable to have skin-to-skin or cuddles then Dad/partner/birthing partner can do so instead.

If you and your baby are separated for a medical reason and you wish to breastfeed, while you may not be able to latch your baby directly to the breast, you can hand-express colostrum (your earliest type of milk) as soon as possible. This is a fantastic way of supporting your colostrum and breast milk supply as well as helping your baby's growth and development, and protecting them from infections through the powerful health properties in your colostrum. If you have been colostrum harvesting, as we talked about in Chapter 4, it is the same technique, but if you are not sure how to do it, do not worry because you will have help on hand in the hospital to support you with this.

FINDING YOUR FEET

There is no normal way to feel when your baby is born. Most new parents question themselves and worry if they are doing a good enough job. Here is the thing: just by thinking this shows you are an incredible parent, and the reality is that, in the eyes of your baby, no one does it better than you – and their opinion far outweighs anyone else's.

As your little one becomes more awake, take time to enjoy eye contact. Although their vision is not very clear at first, they will quickly learn to recognise your face and that will bring them great comfort and calm as they navigate this new world. In fact, tapping into your and your baby's range of senses – smelling them, looking at their little skin folds and tiny fingers and toes, stroking their baby-soft skin – is a great way to bond together. Although you are aware your baby is not still physically a part of you, there is evidence to suggest that they do not realise they are a separate person until around seven months old. This explains why babies love to be close and cuddled and, despite the newborn images you may have seen in the media of babies asleep in cribs, they usually don't like being put down in a crib in those early days. Smelling your baby and allowing them to smell the comfort of you, singing, massaging and chatting away to your little one are all ways of getting to know each other.

It is normal to not love every moment or every feed or even every day of parenthood, and some days do feel a challenge. This is where finding your tribe and having someone who you can share how you are honestly feeling with on those tough days is really helpful.

PAUSE FOR THOUGHT

What would you like your golden hour to look and feel like? Let's plan it. It can be useful to look at all five of your senses here again, just like you did in Chapter 5 with your birth environment planning, and you can add this into your birth preference planner on page 223.

When your baby is born, I encourage you to allow yourself to let a feeling of strength swaddle you, almost like a warm, comforting blanket. Because, whatever the hours or days that came before this moment may have looked like, you did it – you brought your baby into the world and have crossed the bridge into motherhood. This is a moment that needs recognising. Your strength and courage needs celebrating, and the golden hour provides the perfect opportunity to do this. Women are truly incredible.

The next chapter is going to arm you with the essentials you need to care for your newborn baby.

REMEMBER:

- Pause after your baby is born and cherish the experience you have just been through together. Have a real look at their little face, take in their smell and kiss them as much as you wish. You did it!
- Take photos or videos to make precious memories in those earliest moments.
- Embrace skin-to-skin, uninterrupted, for as long as possible and continue to have skin-to-skin over the days and weeks that follow, feeling your baby's breathing and heart rate against yours.

18

CARING FOR YOUR NEWBORN BABY

It is a funny feeling arriving home with your newborn baby. I remember it well – we sat on the sofa with this tiny, beautiful bundle, tucking into a takeaway and, despite having only been a twosome less than 12 hours before this moment, we couldn't remember our lives before our baby's arrival. There was this warm feeling of intense love, but also a sense of responsibility and newness that can be overwhelming.

I think it is fair to say that a degree of mild and manageable anxiety and overwhelm with a new baby is normal. But having an idea of what to expect and how to help your baby in the immediate newborn days will help put your mind at ease and allow you to continue into the journey of the fourth trimester with the same calm confidence with which you approached birth. You should also always know that, although you may be physically on your own, healthcare professionals are still on hand if you are ever worried about your baby. You can always call your midwife, health visitor or GP, or 111 out of hours, and, of course, if you feel you or your baby need urgent medical help, you can phone 999.

I am conscious of not overloading your mind as you prepare for birth and parenthood, but I want to give you enough information so that you feel well-equipped and not taken by total surprise when your baby is finally in your arms. In this chapter, I am going to guide you through some of the essential, immediate newborn care and tips and tricks to help you along the way.

> *These things will be hard to do but you can do hard things.*
>
> Glennon Doyle, *We Can Do Hard Things*

BABY CHECKS AND VITAMIN K

After your golden hour, your baby will have a top-to-toe check, be weighed, have their head circumference measured, temperature checked, and you will be offered vitamin K for your baby.

Vitamin K is offered to all newborn babies in the UK because a small number of babies develop a rare condition called 'vitamin K deficiency bleeding' (VKDB). VKDB can cause serious bleeding so the purpose of supplementing babies with vitamin K is to reduce the risk of VKDB. Early and classical VKDB occurs in 1 in 60 to 1 in 250 newborns. With the appropriate dose and timing of vitamin K supplementation, the likelihood of your baby developing VKDB is reduced to 1 in 100,000. There are two ways to give vitamin K to babies: as an injection into baby's thigh or orally. The main advantage of the injection is it only requires one dose and is more effective at reducing VKDB. However, it does cause temporary pain at the injection site and may leave a small bruise. The oral vitamin K is given in three doses at one day, one week and one month of age. The challenge is it is not possible to know how much baby has absorbed and they are prone to vomiting at this age too.

Most parents do opt to have vitamin K, but it is entirely your choice and you do not have to accept it. If you have concerns over receiving vitamin K, it is important to have a discussion with your medical team to look at the individual protective or risk factors specific to you and your baby.

You will also be offered the newborn and infant physical examination (NIPE), which is part of a screening programme to check newborn babies within 72 hours of birth. This happens again between six and eight weeks for conditions relating to their heart, hips, eyes and testes. You will be told the results straight away and, if there are any concerns, referrals to specialists can be arranged.

NAPPY CHANGING

Having a baby and becoming an expert nappy changer basically come hand in hand. But nappies are more than a messy, smelly nuisance! Your little one's nappies can also provide great reassurance that they are well-hydrated, feeding well and thriving, so it is useful to know what to expect from your baby in terms of urine and stools, and the frequency and colour that is normal.

You will find your household conversations become quite poo-focused in the early days with a new baby; it is the new parents' common dinner table chat. If your baby's poos are changing colour from black to brown/green and mustard and they are having regular wet nappies, this is a great sign that they are doing well and getting enough milk. If your baby's poo is black (after the initial meconium poo is passed), grey, red or white, it could mean there is an underlying health issue, so contact your GP right away.

A NOTE ON TYPES OF NAPPY

We have all seen the conventional disposable nappy, but have you considered reusable cloth nappies? Modern cloth nappies come in a variety of types and are now as easy to put on as a disposable. The big win on cloth nappies is their positive impact on the environment. The government department Defra completed a Lifecycle Assessment comparing the impact of disposable and cloth nappies in 2023 and they found that reusable nappies produce 25 per cent less CO_2 than disposables and the environmental impact of production is over 90 per cent lower for a reusable nappy than for a disposable. Even when factoring in washing and drying, reusable nappies still proved to be the best nappy choice for the environment, with reusables using a huge 97.5 per cent fewer raw materials than disposables. The great thing is there are so many options for reusable nappies now there truly is something to suit any family, and many parents choose to use them part-time so there is no pressure to do all or nothing either. Even if reusable nappies aren't for you, I recommend considering reusable wipes – these are not just amazing for saving plastic wipes in the environment, but are a great money saver for you too. There are some websites in the Further Resources section (page 311) if you want to find more information on these eco swaps.

Changing your baby's nappy regularly is important to stop their skin getting sore and prevent nappy rash; the more sensitive their skin, the quicker their nappy should be changed. Changing your baby's nappy can feel daunting at first and it may take a few changes to get the hang of it as they are so little and wriggly and often cry when their nappy is being changed. Your midwife can guide you through the first nappy or two and a newborn baby will need changing 10–12 times a day, so you really will be an expert in no time.

For girls, it is common that they may have a light bleed from the vagina that can be seen in their nappy – this is nothing to worry about and is the effect of the birth hormones and doesn't last long. Boys' nappy changes come with an extra warning as often the cold air when you undo their dirty nappy causes them to do a wee and, trust me, it goes everywhere! It's a good idea to have something to hand like a small cloth or muslin to contain this. When you've finished changing a boy's nappy, just make sure the penis is facing downwards and not upwards – this will help prevent leaks through the top of their nappy.

Some tips to making sure the nappy is on well include:

- The top of the nappy sits just under baby's belly button (you may need to roll the top down in the early days).
- The leg cuffs run neatly around the top of their thighs. Run your fingers along these to make sure the little frilly bits of fabric aren't tucked inwards.
- You can run two fingers along the waistband when the nappy is done up – this makes sure it isn't too tight. Nappies shouldn't leave any red marks on your baby's skin either. If you notice these, it is a sign the nappy needs to be loosened a little.

Umbilical cord care

There will be a bit of umbilical cord left attached to your baby's belly button after the delivery of your placenta. It usually takes around a week to dry out and drop off. Until this time, you want to keep it as clean and dry as possible to reduce the likelihood of an infection developing. It is normal that the cord goes dark, almost black in colour, as it becomes dry before falling off. If possible, keep the cord out of the nappy to reduce the amount of urine and stool that comes into contact with the cord. Clean and dry it when changing nappies and dry it well after bathing your baby. Should you notice any bleeding, redness or oozing from the site then speak with your midwife, health visitor or GP as this could indicate an infection.

YOUR BABY'S FIRST BATH

Bathing your baby for the first time is such a wonderful moment and memory to treasure, and is often one of the earliest milestones in your parenting journey. It can become a lovely bonding experience and help form part of a bedtime routine which can even incorporate a little bit of baby massage too.

One of the most common questions new parents ask me is when they should give their baby their first bath. It is best not to rush the bath and to wait at least 24 hours – even waiting several days is fine. Babies are born with a special substance on their skin called vernix caseosa, which looks white and waxy, and is wonderful at moisturising your baby's skin. It's good to try to keep this on your baby's skin for as long as possible so, instead of a bath, you can do a 'top and tail' wash where you can simply clean their face, neck, hands and bottom with some warm water and cotton wool or reusable wipes.

Newborn skincare is important to discuss because we often hear conflicting advice and it can be really confusing. The skin is our biggest physical barrier to organisms, providing UV protection, regulating our body temperature and sensory perception. Skin is a complex and dynamic organ, even more so in newborns where is it more sensitive and significantly more absorbent. The challenge for parents is that, despite skin health having a profound impact on their baby's well-being, the regulation around baby-safe products is not as comprehensive as we would hope. The first rule, as discussed above, is to not remove vernix from baby's skin – it is so full of skin goodness, proteins, fatty acids, antimicrobial and antifungal properties that it is your baby's best natural skin protection. Babies who are born past their due date may have drier-looking skin as the vernix has already been absorbed. When our babies are born, their skin pH is higher than adult skin, making it quite alkaline, and this is likely due to exposure to the alkaline amniotic fluid while they are in the womb. In the first few days after birth, the pH level rapidly drops to a more acidic level and forms an 'acid mantle', a protective film on the skin surface that we need to respect and preserve for precious newborn skin. According to recent statistics, around one-third of children will develop eczema, so protecting their skin early on is something to really consider to help reduce the chance of skin complications.

Just because of how important this topic is, I want to share with you some extra newborn skincare information from an expert in this area: Joanna Jensen, founder and CEO of Childs Farm, the UK's number-one baby and child personal care brand:

When our due date approaches, we go through our checklist of purchases: cot, car seat, pram, babygrows, breast pump, and so on, but often baby's skin and hair is left to the last minute or even overlooked. Our skin is the largest organ in our body, and looking after it properly from the very beginning can make a difference in how our skin feels, looks and behaves. Here are my top tips for successful baby skin, as well as some very common skin issues your baby could experience:

Sensitive skin

Take heart in that 1 in 5 under-fives in the UK will suffer from atopic dermatitis – a form of eczema – which is often grown out of by the age of eight. To ease dry, itchy and painful skin, it is important that baby's skin is regularly moisturised with a baby oil or baby moisturiser at least three times a day. Make it part of your routine when getting baby dressed in the morning, at nappy changes and after bath time to keep baby's skin well-nourished. Use a non-bio washing powder for all clothing, nappies and wipes, and use cotton clothes to avoid irritation.

Bathing baby

To prevent irritation, baby's skin needs to be kept clean, and babies can be surprisingly dirty, from milk spills to nappy explosions. During the first month, baby's skin is at its most delicate as it hasn't yet formed the barrier that will eventually protect them from allergens and infection. Most clean-ups can be done topically with some mild baby wash and damp cotton wool or cotton pads.

It is also perfectly safe to bath your baby three times a week from newborn to two months old, but, as their skin is still very thin, don't overdo it. After two months old, bathing can be increased to as often as you both like. Bath water temperature should be warm – no more than 37°C – and kept to no more than five minutes as the water temperature will drop the longer baby is in the bath. You can use a baby bubble bath or baby wash to remove dirt – water on its own will not do this – and baby will love the sensation of bubbles around them too. Use a very soft flannel or cotton pad with water only around baby's eyes to prevent discomfort. Even if your wash maintains it is tear-free, it's better to act on the side of caution. Always support baby's head out of the water with your hand, and never leave baby alone in the bath.

Managing baby's body temperature

One of the main roles of skin is to keep our body temperature regulated and at an even temperature. But your newborn baby's skin isn't yet mature enough to do this and won't be for some months. The surface area of baby's skin versus their weight is three times greater than yours, so baby can lose heat from their body more easily than you. This means that they get hotter or colder more quickly than even a one-year-old. You can help by avoiding extremes of temperature, and that includes bath time.

When you take baby out of the bath, wrap them in a warm towel, pat baby dry and then moisturise their skin all over before getting them *dressed for bed. Keeping a thermometer in baby's bedroom will also allow you to monitor the temperature as they sleep.*

The bum department

Managing baby's bottom cleanliness and moisturisation will prevent all sorts of upset and pain, so follow this three-step guide to success:

1. *Change nappies after every pee or poo.*
2. *Clean off dirt and damp with warm soapy water and a soft cloth. Skin irritation occurs when dirt remains in open pores, so be thorough but gentle.*
3. *After every change, moisturise baby's bum and leg creases with a good nappy cream to seal in moisture and prevent irritation.*

Cradle cap and how to manage it

During pregnancy, your hormones pass through the placenta into your baby's bloodstream. Once they are born, some of these hormones remain in their system and it's these that can be responsible for cradle cap. This is a baby skin condition where thin, waxy white or pale-yellow scales appear on baby's scalp.

While tempting, do resist the urge to pick these scales off. Instead, rub the scalp with a gentle moisturiser designed for babies with sensitive skin to get the loose scales away from the skin. At bath time, massage in a gentle, moisturising baby shampoo and rinse well. Be patient – it will go if just moisturised three or four times a day.

Baby acne

All the hormones that have been passed through to baby in the womb can also manifest themselves in what is called baby acne. This presents as small, red spots usually on the nose and cheeks. These can last from a few weeks old up to four months. Left alone, baby acne should go away. Washing with a mild baby wash will help prevent further irritation and keep the skin clean. Dab a tiny bit on a cotton ball and clean one cheek, then use another cotton ball with plain water to rinse. Repeat on the other cheek.

The first year of baby's skin

It will take 12 months before your baby will have the same skin barrier protection that you have, so it's vital that you spend the time required to keep their skin clean and moisturise to create a good skin barrier.

Managing baby in the sun

As babies' skin has little melanin – the skin's natural sun protector – it's important that they are never exposed to the sun in their first six months, and after that are kept out of direct sunshine as much as possible. UV rays penetrate glass and cloth, so make sure you fit anti-UV sunshades to car windows and invest in anti-UV shades for the pram and cot. As baby grows, they will be in the sun more, so be sure to apply a minimum of 50 SPF on their skin and reapply often. Anti-UV clothes are also available, but use a cream as well.

Swimming and changing

One of the most fun things you can do with your baby is swimming, which helps them feel comfortable in water very early on, and is great for being sociable with other babies. Splashing their face with water in the bath can help them get used to the unpredictable behaviour of water in the swimming baths and the splashing their little peers will generate too. After swimming, bring an all-in-one wash/shampoo solution for the shower so you're not trying to juggle baby and bottles. It's important you wash off the chlorine from baby's skin as soon as possible, so a single bottle will make life a lot easier, and you can also use it for yourself too.

FEEDING YOUR BABY

However you choose to feed your baby, the most important thing is you can feed them with love and in a way that feels right for you; this may be breastfeeding exclusively, combination feeding (breast-feeding and bottle-feeding with either expressed breast milk or infant formula milk), or bottle-feeding with formula milk.

Breastfeeding

It is probably not brand-new news to hear that breastfeeding has a whole heap of benefits for both you and your baby, so this may feel like a little recap, but there may also be some surprise benefits you hadn't heard of.

Let's start off with some of the benefits for baby:

- Helps to protect your baby from infections, as breast milk contains immune factors.
- Straight after birth and for the first few days of breastfeeding, your breast milk contains colostrum, which is full of antibodies that help protect your baby from infections.
- Continuing breastfeeding is important to make sure your baby will benefit from the antibodies in your breast milk on an ongoing basis. As you come into contact with new infections, your baby will automatically get some immunity from them too.
- Helps your baby become a lifelong healthy eater – as your breast milk is uniquely tailored to your baby and, incredibly, the food you eat while breastfeeding can influence their taste preferences throughout weaning and beyond.
- Helps reduce your baby's chances of having diarrhoea or vomiting.
- Helps reduce the risk of the following health complications for your baby: sudden infant death syndrome (SIDS), type 2 diabetes and childhood leukaemia.

- Helps reduce the risk of diseases later in life, including: cardiovascular disease, eczema, asthma and other allergies, and obesity.
- It lines your baby's gut with healthy gut bacteria or microbiota, which continues to protect your little one from illness and infection. It literally supports your baby's healthier future.

And for mum, it is also a whole lotta goodness:

- Helps you to lose any weight gained during pregnancy, as you burn approximately 500 extra calories a day while exclusively breastfeeding, BUT remember, while your body is recovering, it is important to supplement this calorie deficit with nutritional food.
- Helps to strengthen the bond between you and your baby.
- Holding your baby while they're feeding provides intimacy through skin-to-skin contact. This closeness comforts your baby while helping to regulate their heart rate and body temperature.
- Lowers your chances of postpartum depression.
- Lowers your chances of ovarian and breast cancer.
- Saves you preparation time – as there's no need to sterilise bottles and other feeding preparation.
- Saves you money on formula, bottles and preparation equipment.

A few extra surprising facts for you:

- Your breast milk is totally unique to you – its composition is shaped by your diet, hormones, genetics, environmental influences and the individual needs of you and your baby.
- Your baby recognises the smell of your breast milk – the scent of your breast milk prompts your newborn to show searching behaviours.

- Your breast milk contains calming sleepy hormones which help your baby to sleep.
- Breast milk is different for sons and daughters: boys consume more of their mother's milk than girls and, amazingly, the breast milk produced for boys contains 25 per cent more calories than for girls.

So there we have it: your milk is your Mumma superpower!

Breastfeeding is a skill that you and your baby learn together, and it can take time to get used to. Getting off to a good start with positioning and attaching your baby to the breast can really help prevent issues such as nipple damage and excessive baby weight loss from arising.

HOW TO LATCH YOUR BABY ON TO YOUR BREAST

1. Hold your baby close to you with their nose level with your nipple.
2. Let your baby's head tip back a little so that their top lip can brush against your nipple. This should help your baby to make a wide, open mouth.
3. When your baby's mouth is open wide enough, their chin should be able to touch your breast first, with their head tipped back so that their tongue can reach as much of your breast as possible.
4. With your baby's chin firmly touching your breast and their nose clear, their mouth should be wide open. When they attach you should see much more of the darker nipple skin above your baby's top lip than below their bottom lip. Your baby's cheeks will look full and rounded as they feed.

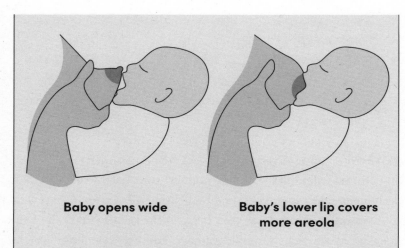

Baby opens wide   **Baby's lower lip covers more areola**

It is important that your baby has a good mouthful of breast to ensure they are effectively getting milk and to protect your nipple. If you run your tongue over the roof of your mouth you will notice your palate is hard and ridged at the front and soft at the back. Your baby's mouth is the same, so you want to ensure your nipple is on the soft area.

If your baby doesn't appear to be latched well, it is important you readjust to prevent complications. To take baby off the breast without damaging your nipple, simply pop your little finger in the side of their mouth to break the seal they have on the nipple and then guide them off.

A good latch is also key to help prevent engorgement and blocked ducts. It is important to try to prevent and treat these early as they may become infected and lead to a common breastfeeding problem called mastitis. Mastitis causes swelling and inflammation, so may make you feel like you have tender breasts. You are also likely to feel achy, run-down and feverish; and you may have flu-like symptoms. If you suspect you have mastitis, please speak with your GP as you may need antibiotics. It is important for your baby to continue breastfeeding to help prevent the infection from turning into an abscess.

As you and your baby learn the new skill of breastfeeding, some mothers will experience nipple damage, pain and new sensations as baby latches and you feel the let-down reflex of milk for the first few times. All of this can feel new and sensitive, but, over time, things will settle – you will both get the hang of it and it will become easier. It is really important you seek expert support from your midwife, health visitor or trained breastfeeding practitioner to ensure that what you're feeling is normal and is not a sign of a latch issue or tongue tie.

Leaking breasts are common in the early days and weeks of feeding. My postman was greeted by big milk rings on my top more times than I care to confess, alongside the odd time I forgot to readjust my feeding bra and top and had a boob out too! Breast pads really are an essential, and changing them regularly helps prevent skin infections developing. Over time, as your milk supply regulates, the leaking will settle, so hang on in there and pack a spare T-shirt for you as well as baby in the first few months if you're out and about.

A breastfed baby that feeds very regularly or 'cluster feeds' is not a sign that your milk supply isn't sufficient – it is a normal pattern of behaviour and supports establishing your milk supply for the longer term. If you want to breastfeed, try not to worry about not having enough milk. It is truly very rare for women to not have enough milk. The issue is usually around understanding newborn behaviour and feeding expectations. Gather your support and advice army from the get-go. I've included some helpful breastfeeding resources in the Further Resources (page 311): The Breastfeeding Network and UNICEF are both worth checking out.

Breastfeeding positions

There are lots of different positions you can use to breastfeed. You can try different ones to find out what works best for you and your little one. The four most common breastfeeding positions are:

1. **Cradle hold:** If you've had a caesarean, this may be uncomfortable as your baby lies across your tummy near the scar. Make sure you are well-supported with pillows/cushions. Having a little stool/cushion under your feet will also help support your back and posture in this position.

2. **Side-lying:** This is a good position if you've had a caesarean and can also be nice when you're breastfeeding in the middle of the night.

3. **Laid-back nursing:** Also known as 'biological nursing', this is when you lie back in a semi-reclined position on a comfy sofa or bed. This position can be a lovely way to introduce some early tummy time to your baby.

4. **Rugby ball:** The rugby hold is a good position for twins as you can feed them at the same time, as well as caesarean babies as there's no pressure on the scar area. For women with larger breasts it can allow you to see your baby and check their latch easier.

Below are some pointers to run through when your baby is on the breast to check your positioning:

- Are you comfortable? It's worth making sure you're comfortable before a feed. Use pillows or cushions if necessary. Your shoulders and arms should be relaxed.
- Are your baby's head and body in a straight line? It's hard for your baby to swallow if their head and neck are twisted.

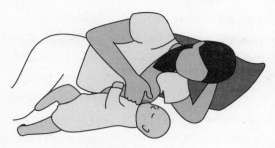

Side-lying

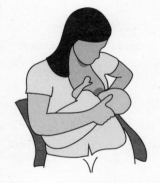

Cross-cradle hold

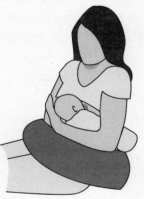

Laid-back nursing

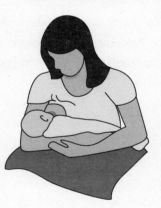

Cradle hold

Rugby ball hold

- Are you holding your baby close to you, facing your breast? Supporting their neck, shoulders and back should allow them to tilt their head back and swallow easily.
- Always bring your baby to the breast and let them latch themselves. Avoid leaning your breast forward into your baby's mouth, as this can lead to poor attachment.
- Your baby needs to get a big mouthful of breast – check their latch (see page 255).
- Try not to hold the back of your baby's head, so that they can tip their head back.

The acronym CHINS can help you to remember these pointers:

- Close
- Head free
- In line
- Nose to nipple
- Sustainable

Signs your baby is getting enough milk

A number one worry for breastfeeding mums is how to know their baby is getting enough milk when they can't actually see the volume. But it is reassuring to know there are a number of ways by which you can do this:

- Your baby starts feeding with a few rapid sucks followed by longer sucks.
- Their cheeks stay rounded out, not sucked in, and you can hear them swallowing.
- Your baby seems calm during feeding and comes off your breast themselves when they've had enough.
- They appear content and satisfied after most feeds.

- They should be healthy and gaining weight (although it's normal for babies to lose a little weight in the first week after birth).
- After the first few days, your baby should have at least six wet nappies a day.
- After about five days, your baby's poo should stop looking black and thick, and they should also have at least two soft or runny yellow poos per day.

BREAST CHANGES

Breastfeeding mums may also notice breast changes. Especially as colostrum turns into mature milk, your breasts will, often quite suddenly, become larger and full. They can feel hard and engorged until you feed. This is normal and regular feeding is the quickest, simplest way to help your body regulate your supply and improve your comfort.

Bottle-feeding

The first thing to note about bottle-feeding your baby is that taking time to have skin-to-skin either during a bottle-feed or just for a cuddle is a great way to promote bonding and help your little one to regulate their temperature and heart rate. Your new baby will usually feel more secure when the majority of their bottle-feeds are given by their caregivers in the early days and weeks. Looking at your baby, singing or talking to them while feeding them their bottle can also form an important part of your bonding.

Formula milk is usually made from cows' milk which is treated to make it more suitable for babies and has added vitamins. There are some different types of formula available and it is important to check the packaging to make sure you're buying first infant formula (first milk) for your newborn baby. The reason for this is that the cows' milk in formula contains two types of protein: whey and casein. Whey is thought to be easier to digest and is typically found in first infant formula. This milk also contains the appropriate vitamin doses for new babies.

Let me walk you through how to correctly bottle-feed your baby:

- Hold your baby semi-upright and close to you, and gently invite them to open their mouth by rubbing the bottle teat against their upper lip.
- Then, when your baby is ready, gently pop the teat into their mouth with the bottle slightly tipped in a horizontal position. This helps to stop milk flowing too quickly and is a gentler way to bottle-feed.
- During a feed, watch your baby and respond to them showing signs of needing a pause. They may do things like splaying their fingers, spilling milk out of their mouth, turning their head away, pushing the bottle away, or they may simply stop sucking. If you notice these cues, you can remove the bottle and pause the feed while they have a little break. Your baby may need a few little breaks and will need burping during and after a feed.

Some equipment you will need to bottle-feed your baby includes: several bottles, teats and a bottle brush, as well as sterilising equipment (you can use cold-water, microwave or steam sterilisers).

You should be careful to wash your hands before making up a bottle and it is advised to make up each feed fresh so that bacteria can't grow and cause your little one to become unwell. The infant formula you buy will have manufacturer instructions and it is important to follow these, avoiding adding any extra powder as this can lead to constipation and dehydration for babies.

TONGUE TIE

Tongue ties are often undiagnosed and can be really challenging in the early days of feeding. If you suspect this might be the problem, discuss this with your midwife, health visitor or GP, and, if available to you, look for a trained private practitioner to assess your baby.

Combination feeding

It doesn't have to be all-or-nothing when it comes to breastfeeding your baby – you can also choose to combine breast- and bottle-feeding. However, it is best to establish breastfeeding and ensure you and your baby are confident with it before adding in a bottle. Your bottle could contain expressed breast milk or formula milk. It is important to do this process gradually and gently to allow time for your breasts and milk supply to adapt and help prevent engorgement, mastitis (see page 256) or milk supply issues. It may also take some time for your baby to get used to a bottle as it is a very different feeding technique for them than from the breast, so being gentle, patient and reassuring is helpful. Some parents find combination feeding provides a helpful balance to give the breast-feeding mum a break or time to rest.

FEEDING CUES

With all types of feeding, you want to feed your baby when they show signs of being hungry. You can do this by looking out for their feeding cues, such as facial movements, moving their head and mouth around, stretching and sucking on their fingers or fist. Crying is the last sign of wanting to feed, so try to feed your baby before they cry (this isn't always possible, but, as your baby grows and you get to know them better, it does become easier). As you observe and get to know your baby more, their feeding cues become more obvious, so don't worry if you miss these at first.

When bottle-feeding your baby it is advised to do this responsively, which means watching and responding to their feeding cues, offering the bottle in a gentle way and watching them as they feed, responding to signs they may wish to have a pause or stop.

WINDING YOUR BABY

Winding or burping your baby goes hand in hand with feeding. When your baby swallows during a feed, air bubbles become trapped in their stomach and cause discomfort. Some babies find it easy to burp up these troublesome bubbles themselves, while others may need a little help. And just like us adults, some babies are windier than others. If you are breastfeeding, it's important to ensure your baby has a good seal around the breast, which will help to reduce their intake of air while feeding, reducing issues with wind and digestive discomfort.

Some babies are naturally windier than others and may need winding during and after a feed. If your baby appears uncomfortable during a feed, it is a good idea to stop to burp them, and always burp at the end of a feed too. Usually for a breastfed baby winding at the end of a feed is sufficient. A few pointers to help you with burping your little one are to ensure you always support their head and neck, and make sure that their tummy and back are straight rather than curled up. Then it is simply a case of gently rubbing or patting their back gently. There are many positions such as over your shoulder, sitting on your lap or lying across your lap, and it is just a case of seeing which is most effective for your little one.

It is always a good idea to have a muslin cloth nearby when burping your baby as they often bring up a little milk when they burp. This is really normal and not something to worry about, but save your clothes by being prepared.

Scan the QR code on page 6 for a demonstration of some of these burping positions.

NEW BABY SLEEP

Honestly, if you checked out my most searched terms when I first became a mum they would have all been about newborn sleep. The reality is new babies have no idea about the difference between day-time and night-time and they have found themselves in this very odd new world that is completely different to the life they knew inside you. There are strange sounds, lights and noises, the temperature fluctuates, they are wearing clothing that feels different on their skin . . . All of this newness can feel overwhelming to a new baby and, as parents, you are their safe space while they learn (and they will in time) to navigate this new environment. They haven't yet figured out what their arms and legs are doing and often wake themselves up with these moving limbs they find attached to them. What they love is being snuggled up close to their parents where they feel warm and safe and can smell you and hear your familiar heart rate. I think as new parents when we can put ourselves in the shoes of our new baby and try to understand what they are feeling, it can make new baby sleep a calmer journey for all.

When we picture a new baby, we no doubt imagine a perfect little bundle cosily tucked up in a cot or Moses basket sleeping. And all the images online don't help with this idealised picture. What you will not see is how long it took their parent to get them there. Some babies take to being placed down to sleep well; most, however, would much rather have that reassuring cuddle, so settling them into cots can be a challenge. I cannot tell you the amount of times I have placed my son down and ninja'd out of the room – let me tell you, it is a skill.

When you think about your baby's environment inside you, it is useful to try to replicate some of this in their sleep space to help them soothe and settle. For example, you can sleep with their cot sheet down your top before you use it so it smells of you, pre-warm their sheet so it isn't a shock in winter months that it feels colder than your arms (a hot water bottle in the cot before placing baby in works well, but of course check it isn't too hot and remove it before putting your baby in). Lots of babies also love the sound of white noise. We forget the sounds that your baby is used to hearing in the womb aren't quite what they will hear in the outside world – the whooshing sound of the placenta and blood flow, as well as your heartbeat. That's why the classic 'shhhh, shhhh, shhhh' works so well for babies and a white noise sound that matches that can help calm them. There are lots of white noise machines on the market and my husband and I cannot sleep without one – it is so restful for your mind. Dimmed or dark lighting reduces stimulation and can also help babies to settle. Over time you can begin to help them differentiate between day and night with lots of bright light in awake times and darker lighting in sleep or night-times.

> Every parent's sleep journey is different and every baby is so unique in their sleep needs and patterns.

A newborn will have no definitive routine, so roll with it and, if you can, embrace the flexibility. I remember going on a walking and pub dinner holiday when our little boy was eight weeks old and I am so grateful we did. At the time, it felt like it would be a challenge because we were tired new parents, but in reality we wouldn't be able to do that again because, as babies get older, they tend to need routine, so you can't so easily sit with them asleep in a carrier at 10pm tucking into pub food by a roaring fire. Every stage of your parenting journey will have its own challenges and its own advantages, but know that, even in the most difficult moments, it is only a phase and it will pass with easier days ahead.

I am not going to tell you to 'sleep when the baby sleeps' because, although for some new mums this is achievable – and if it is please embrace it because sleep is a priority in the early weeks – for many it is not realistic. You may have other children to care for, you may not have the physical support of family and friends nearby, you may have work commitments or you may just need some time to be: to shower, to eat a hot meal with two hands, to do something for you. So instead of 'sleep when the baby sleeps', my advice is to simply get rest in when you can – a bit like you would put your phone on charge when the battery is low, you need to recharge your body too.

If I have one regret of my motherhood journey it would be the pressure and expectations I put on sleep that didn't serve us and caused unnecessary stress, because the reality was our little boy was going to feed to sleep and enjoy a contact nap whether I got anxious about it or not. I don't want you to fall into the sleep comparison and pressure trap I fell into the first time around, so I have some expert tips from Rosey Davidson, sleep consultant and author of *The Just Chill Baby Sleep Book*, here for you:

Sleep is one of those topics that everyone talks about. Most parents (if not all!) will struggle with it at some point. For many people, having a newborn can be the first time in their lives when they have ever experienced sleep deprivation.

The first three months of a baby's life, often referred to as the fourth trimester, are a period of significant adjustment for both the infant and their parents. Understanding what is normal for newborns can be really helpful. While each baby is individual, it is very normal for them to wake often and need reassurance or input from their parents to get to sleep. This could be feeding, rocking, swaying, bouncing or safe bed sharing.

Babies in their first three months of life have not yet developed mature sleep patterns and, as a result, their sleep is often fragmented and unpredictable. It can be helpful and comforting to know that this disruption is entirely normal and expected during the fourth trimester.

During this time, babies typically sleep for short periods, waking frequently to feed, be changed or simply seek comfort. This pattern can be really exhausting, but it will pass. These frequent awakenings are a survival mechanism, ensuring that newborns get the nourishment and care they need to grow and thrive. It is also really normal for them to want to be close to their caregivers.

Caring for a newborn during the fourth trimester can be overwhelming, especially for first-time parents. It's therefore crucial to build a support network to help navigate this challenging period. Friends, family members or even professional support, such as a sleep consultant, health visitor or lactation consultant, can offer valuable guidance and assistance.

Accepting help and delegating tasks when possible can reduce stress and allow you to get much-needed rest. Remember, it takes a village to raise a child, and there's no shame in seeking support to ensure your baby's well-being and your own mental and physical health.

While the fourth trimester may be a time of disrupted sleep, it's never too early to start laying the foundation for healthy sleep habits. One thing we can focus on is helping your baby distinguish between day and night.

During the day, expose your baby to natural light. Natural light helps regulate the body's internal clock, or circadian rhythm, which controls sleep–wake cycles. When your baby is exposed to daylight, it helps them learn that daytime is for alertness and play, while night-time is for rest.

Keep night-time interactions with your baby calm and subdued. Avoid bright lights and stimulating activities. When your baby wakes at night for feeding or nappy changes, do these tasks quietly and gently, so that you can all get back to sleep as quickly as possible.

Every baby is unique, and there is no one-size-fits-all approach to sleep during the fourth trimester (or beyond). While some babies may naturally begin sleeping for longer stretches, others may take more time to develop more predictable sleep patterns.

Parents should be patient and flexible, adapting to their baby's needs while also gradually introducing routines that promote better sleep. This might include establishing a soothing bedtime routine, creating a comfortable sleep environment and recognising your baby's individual sleep cues. Remember that, with time, sleep patterns will evolve and improve.

Safer sleeping

The final thing I want to encourage you to consider around your new baby is safer sleeping and reducing the risk of SIDS. Safer sleeping is something to plan for as you prepare for your parenthood journey, and having the most up-to-date information to practise safer sleeping techniques saves lives.

Safer sleeping advice aims to reduce the risk of SIDS in babies, often called cot death. This is obviously something no expectant parent wants to think about, but by informing yourself correctly you can help protect your baby.

Below is some key guidance around safer sleeping practice. I would recommend looking at The Lullaby Trust website (see Further Resources, page 311) for lots more information on this topic.

- When we think of sleep, we often think of the night-time, but, when it comes to your new baby, it is important to practise safer sleeping during daytime sleep too.

- The position your baby sleeps in is important – you should always place your newborn baby on their back to sleep and not on their front or side. They should also have their feet at the bottom of their cot or Moses basket so that they can't wriggle down and under any bedding.

- Keep your baby in their cot with just their sheets or blankets and nothing extra that could be pulled over their face or cause an accident. Soft, raised surfaces such as pods, nests, bumpers and pillows should be avoided as they make it harder for your baby to cool down and may make it difficult for your baby to breathe.

- The safest place for your baby to sleep day or night is in a cot in the same room as you or their carer for the first six months. This may be a cot (next-to-me-style or standalone), Moses basket, crib, carry cot or travel cot, so have a think about how this will logistically work for you in your home and lifestyle set-up.

- Your baby should sleep on a firm, flat mattress with a waterproof cover – this allows you to keep the mattress clean and dry. Your mattress should ideally be new and should fit the cot or Moses basket properly.

- Keep your baby's sheets and blankets below shoulder height and tuck them in firmly. Avoid using bulky loose bedding such as quilts and duvets. A baby sleeping bag can be a great option as long as it is the correct size and tog for your baby and season, and you do not need to use any other bedding if you are using a sleeping bag. Always follow the product guidelines on the appropriate age and temperature range for your baby's sleeping bag.

- It is important to try to avoid your baby getting too hot or too cold. To check their temperature, feel your baby's chest and/ or back of their neck to ensure their skin doesn't feel too hot, clammy or sweaty to the touch. Babies do not need to wear a hat indoors. They may have done so if they were born in hospital, but once they are home this can cause them to overheat. An ideal room temperature is 16–20°C. A room thermometer can be really useful for helping you judge the temperature in the room where your baby sleeps. You can help keep your baby's room cooler by using blackout blinds and a fan (not directly on your baby). You can also adjust the clothing and layers on your baby depending on the room temperature.

- Breastfeeding has also been shown to reduce the risk of SIDS (SIDS risk is halved in babies who are breastfed for at least two months).

- Smoking during pregnancy and in the postpartum is known to greatly increase the risk of SIDS. Stopping smoking can really help reduce your baby's risk of SIDS and the less you smoke the less risk they are at. If you do smoke it is not advisable to co-sleep with your baby.

I totally understand that SIDS is not something you may want to think about, but by considering some of these simple tips you can really reduce the risk to your little one.

One thing I wish I knew the first time that I had a newborn was just how resilient they are. I've spent the last three months doing two under two. My little one has been sat on, bitten, poked, hit (and given lots of kisses!) by her big sister. I've missed naps and feeding cues, left her in a dirty nappy too long and with sick all down her front. And she's thriving! I guess I would have just told myself more the first time that I won't always get the little things right. As long as a newborn has somewhere safe to sleep and live, and is cared for the best you can manage, they'll be just fine.

Alice

PAUSE FOR THOUGHT

I know newborn care can feel like information overload, and overwhelm at the responsibility can creep in, so here is your space to consider your thoughts. What is most important to you and your family and what is the key newborn care you will be considering or implementing for your baby?

Most new parents feel a sense of overwhelm when they arrive home with their new baby – you are now responsible for this new, precious little life and, naturally, you want to get everything right. The truth is, there is a lot of learning on the job and there is no one right or wrong way to parent. You will become the expert in your baby and what works for your friends or family may not work for you, so know it is OK to find your own way to do things. And remember, you can refer back to this chapter as much as you need to when your little one is here.

Naturally, caring for your new baby takes priority when they arrive, but we must remember that mums matter too, and the next chapter is designed to recognise exactly that.

REMEMBER:

- Take your time to adjust to life as a parent, getting to know your baby and the new responsibilities that come with this.
- Trust that on hard days better days are coming – everything is just a phase that passes.
- If you are ever worried about your newborn baby, call your midwife, health visitor or GP. If you are concerned about your baby's breathing or feel they need urgent medical help, phone 999.

19

SUPPORTING YOUR MENTAL WELL-BEING

Birth and motherhood are not just physical, but are also huge psychological events. We delve into physical changes in the next chapter, but we are kicking off with your mental well-being as this is often the most overlooked. The common phrase 'who is looking after the mum?' is so valid, because you too have just been born into motherhood and are learning at a rapid rate about this new role and identity, you have a small person (or persons) who is entirely dependent on you, you are navigating sleep deprivation and a body that feels very different . . . It can all feel overwhelming, and it is normal to experience a vast range of emotions during this time, especially given the hormonal rollercoaster that your body also goes on post-birth.

This topic deserves its own book as it is a huge subject with so many variables and, thankfully, it is something we are getting better at learning about and lifting the lid on. The reality is that it is often those closest to a new mum who recognise signs of mental health deterioration, and, because of this, I recommend you ask your partner, mum, sister, best friend or whoever is going to be around, to have a read of this chapter too.

Mental health conditions, such as anxiety and depression, are very common. Around 1 in 5 women will develop a mental health condition in pregnancy or within one year postpartum, though it's worth remembering that there is a wide range of severity and impact when it comes to mental health. We do know, however, that many women suffer in silence, so these statistics are likely to be higher than the actual numbers. The purpose of this chapter is to help you recognise what is and is not normal, to explore some of the whirlwind of feelings you may experience and to ensure you know that there is support available. And, most importantly, that asking for help is not a sign of weakness, but it is you getting treatment in the same way you would do if you broke your arm – it is a necessity and the sooner help is started the better. Some women worry that speaking up about their mental health will mean their baby is removed from their care. I want to reassure you this is not the case and seeking support and help is a really good sign that you want to protect your baby and be the best mum to them, so it will never reflect badly on you as a parent.

'I let go of my fear and stay centred in the moment.'

THE BABY BLUES

During the first few weeks following giving birth, up to 80 per cent of women experience a phase called the baby blues. I remember this feeling well as I sat in my nursing chair and felt a sudden flood of tears fall over my exhausted face and overwhelmed body. It is, in a nutshell, a temporary period of low mood at a time when you are expecting to feel super happy, and is thought to be due to the sudden hormonal and chemical changes that occur in a woman's body after giving birth. Women experiencing baby blues may feel more anxious or restless, feel teary for no apparent reason, be irritable and have a low mood, but it should only last a few days before passing. Talking about and monitoring baby blues is important to ensure you notice early if it persists or turns into something more. If you are pondering over whether it is time to ask for help, in my experience it usually is, and it is much better to ask for support early on – this could be from friends or family or a professional, such as your midwife, health visitor or GP. It can be helpful to journal each day following birth if you feel low, even just with very basic words or how your mood is on a scale of 1 to 10, so that you can keep track of how long these feelings last. I have included a mood diary for the first six weeks post-birth on page 308 for you to fill in. I cannot recommend enough taking a minute or two each day to check in with this diary.

POSTNATAL ANXIETY

Anxiety can have a huge spectrum from mild to severe and it is something that professional help can support you to manage. A degree of anxiety as you navigate this new role of motherhood and the responsibilities that come with caring for your new baby is common and some worry is natural. But a constant, uncontrollable feeling of worry about your baby and a persistent feeling of being on edge is a sign that you would benefit from some help and support.

Adopting calming tools such as affirmations or breathing techniques like your upwards breath for birth (see page 47) can help to calm a racing mind in an outburst of anxiety. There are also some tips for managing anxiety from psychotherapist and bestselling author Anna Mathur on page 281. Often, in the fast-paced world we live in, we can trigger anxious feelings because we are worrying over future events that may not even happen – this is very true in motherhood. Often mums find themselves wondering whether they are doing something right, why their baby isn't doing something their friend's baby is or constantly checking their baby is breathing when they are asleep. Try to remain grounded in the present and to not let your mind wander off too far into future issues that may never be a problem for you. If you do find these anxious thoughts are becoming increasingly present, you should seek support: in the Further Resources section (page 311) I have included a link to Mind, which is a great mental health charity.

POSTNATAL DEPRESSION

Postnatal depression (PND) is different to baby blues, and women with PND require professional medical support. PND is thought to affect around 1 in 10 women, which is why it is so important we talk about it and don't give in to it being a taboo subject. This only causes many women to suffer in silence and this should never be the case.

PND typically occurs two to eight weeks after the birth, though it can happen anytime in the year post-birth. I have added a link to a PND awareness and support charity – PANDAS – in the Further Resources (page 311), which has great information for anyone affected by perinatal mental health.

Signs and symptoms of PND to look out for, or to ask someone close to you to observe, are:

- constant crying
- lack of enjoyment in anything
- persistent feelings that you can't cope or of hopelessness
- inability to concentrate and memory loss
- excessive worry and anxiety over the baby
- inability to bond with or lack of interest in the baby
- insomnia
- panic attacks
- appetite loss
- general feeling of being unwell, aches and pains in the body

Raising your hand to ask for help from your midwife, health visitor or GP, or asking someone close to speak for you, is more important than I can express on this page if you suspect PND. It is really important we recognise that PND is not a sign that you're a bad mother or are unable to cope, and we need to break the stigma and allow women to access the incredible services available to heal their minds and thrive in motherhood.

COMPARISON

A trap that I fell into myself as a new mum, and I repeatedly hear from other new mums, is comparing your journey to others'. Your postnatal body, your baby's sleep, your baby's developmental milestones, your return to work . . . There are so many firsts and new experiences in this time and you, and your baby, will do this journey at your own pace that will be different to those around you. The images of new mums and babies is unavoidable and you will be flooded with it all, as well as well-meaning advice and information, but I urge you to consume it with caution because appearances can be deceiving – there is often a lot more going on behind the smiley new-mum selfies. Comparison is the thief of joy, as they say. I would have shed a lot fewer tears if I had managed to pivot back on to my own path instead of trying to tread on someone else's.

CARING FOR YOU

Caring for yourself and your mind as a mum can fall to the bottom of the priority pile, but I promise you this is not a sustainable way to live and eventually overwhelm leads to burnout. Making small steps to practise self-care is an important part of caring for your mental well-being, both pre- and postnatally.

Self-care doesn't mean eating on the go or a speedy shower – these are basic human needs and acts of self-respect. Self-care is something that nourishes your soul, and brings you calm and joy: a leisurely long bath with your favourite bubbles and candle instead of the two-minute dunk in and out of the shower, for example. It may only be for a short time each day to start with or little snippets of self-care exercises dotted throughout your day, and that's OK, but factor it in as a priority and feel no guilt. Meet a friend for a coffee, get that daily fresh air, prioritise delicious easy meals, accept that offer of help or, even better, ask for it and remember those chores can always wait.

You will very likely find yourself spending a lot of time checking that your baby has the right clothing for the weather outside, is adequately hydrated and has had enough interaction or rest each day. When in this cycle, I urge you to just take note of whether *you* have met these needs for yourself too.

This phase is not forever. Although the days feel long when you're in them, the weeks, months and years that follow are so short.

FINDING YOUR VILLAGE

I want to take a moment to just talk about the concept of the village or tribe in the postpartum because you may, like me, find yourself wondering when this helpful village is going to arrive. We live in a time when many of us have moved away from friends or family, and so you may not have close people around you to help out – and that can feel tough, lonely even. The truth is, we need a village, but we may need to be imaginative as to where that village comes from and recognise that support comes in many different forms.

Your village could consist of hired or paid help, if this is available to you – a cleaner, dog walker or meal delivery service, for example, to lessen the load. Or your village may come in a virtual or online form from community groups, social media or texting and calling friends. Having a social media presence was so helpful for me in the postpartum because if I posted about a rough night or a societal pressure, I would be inundated with messages from others going through the same. It made me realise that the more we share our realities within like-minded communities, the more we build an incredible virtual village of support. Texting other new mums in the night who are also up feeding their baby made my nights a lot more bearable and a lot less dark and lonely. Your village may even crop up in the form of strangers through attending local groups. Searching local baby massage, breastfeeding, baby sensory, baby library or buggy walking groups, for example, will lead you to a direct, local community of other new parents navigating the same journey and the same challenges as you.

The emotions of motherhood

Away from specific conditions such as anxiety or PND, there is a whole roller coaster of emotions that may crop up in the hours, days, weeks and months that follow the birth of your baby – from anger to a level of love that terrifies you; from eye-stinging exhaustion to pride that makes your heart burst; from overwhelm to a warm sense of contentment. Boredom, a sense of losing yourself and feeling overstimulated are also ways that new mums can find themselves feeling, and there should be no shame in these sensations – they are like little red flags to your mind and body, and if they are cropping up regularly then the chances are your self-care needs are not being fulfilled. This is where taking a pause to recognise what you need to help you manage your thoughts and feelings and how you can achieve this is essential.

Mum guilt is one of the most talked about emotions, and it seems to be relentlessly resting on our shoulders as we move through the stages of motherhood. The reality is, it may always linger and we need to be able to manage it. Often guilt appears as a result of us managing the needs of our life and we are very critical about ourselves, almost bullying in fact. When you feel a sense of guilt about something, imagine what you would say to or how you would advise a friend or someone you love who was feeling this way. The chances are you would respond very differently and the reality is you deserve that level of compassion too.

A boiling up of challenging emotions may lead to more clinical mental health illness, so it is important we recognise, validate and address difficult emotions as they arise. For example, there may be days (or nights) when your baby wants to be held by you and only you, and this may be unavoidable at the time and lead to you feeling 'touched out' (this is a feeling I didn't understand until I became a mum and I quickly began to understand it very well – it is a frustrated, overwhelming feeling of the high demand for people (your newborn most likely) to be physically touching you). Recognise how you feel, communicate it and take an action to help you address this feeling – can you call in some help and go for a 15-minute walk on your own that day, or hibernate in the bath perhaps? I found after a night of constant feeding, a warm shower with my favourite playlist allowed me to wash away any frustrated emotions from the night before and to take on the day with a fresh start.

> *Collect any friends you have who have young children. They've been there. Don't be afraid to message them in the middle of the night. They will reassure you that they've felt the exact same as you have. They'll remind you about the fourth trimester, speak of feeding stories with you, understand the lack of sleep and help you realise your main job right now is cuddling, feeding and raising a baby, not the housework!*
>
> Alysha

As a new parent, it is OK to feel emotions that perhaps you didn't expect to or haven't felt before, because you haven't walked this path before – life after birth is different and our minds are challenged. The more we can speak openly and share the range of emotions of motherhood, the better supported new mums will be.

Below are some top tips from Anna Mathur, psychotherapist and bestselling author:

> *Get good at accepting help, both big and small. So, if someone offers to make you a cup of tea in your own home and everything in you wants to say no, just really challenge yourself to let them. Allow people to do things for you even if it feels uncomfortable. Feel the guilt and do it anyway because the better you become at accepting support with the small things before your baby arrives, the easier you will find it when you really need it.*
>
> *We can often invalidate our emotions and place a lot of pressure on ourselves to feel grateful and happy all of the time, when actually a lot of new motherhood and late pregnancy is exhausting and overwhelming. We*

can very easily say, 'I feel very overwhelmed, but I am really grateful'. I encourage you to change 'but' to 'and'. Try, 'I feel very overwhelmed and I am really grateful' instead. This adds more balance instead of feeling shame over the conflicting emotions you may feel. It is OK to find hard things hard and that doesn't mean you aren't grateful or it's a statement about how much you love your child.

Intrusive thoughts are common and say nothing about who you are or the love you have for your child, they are just your mind playing with risk and responsibility and power and possibility. When we are tired, those things are often harder to rationalise, so notice those thoughts and let them go. Don't allow your mind to turn a thought from 2D words on a page to a full technicolour 4D theatre. If you do experience regular thoughts that are upsetting to you, then get support.

Don't just accept anxiety – you deserve more than anxiety being the background buzz to motherhood, and there is so much that can help, like simple techniques to interrupt rumination such as counting back from 100 in threes, using the birthing breath to calm your fight-or-flight response, or using simple mantras like 'I am safe, I am loved, my baby is safe, my baby is loved.'

Always try to go beyond 'I am OK, I am fine.' Have two or three people in your life who get more than that, who you can be open and honest with about how you are feeling.

Mum guilt will crop up and you will find yourself questioning everything, but your mental health is of upmost priority because if you are OK then the side effect of that is that your baby will benefit. So put your mental health first in whatever decisions you make. We often second-guess ourselves and worry about how other people will judge us, so a good tool is to think: What would I do if no one knew? How would I choose to birth my baby if no one ever knew? How would I feed my baby if no one ever knew? This allows you to get to the core of what is right for you and avoids your decision-making being based on people-pleasing.

It is so easy to push people away when we are having a hard time. I remember messaging a friend saying 'don't come over, I am a mess' but challenged myself to delete don't and say instead, 'come over, I am a mess'. Often, we want people in our homes when everything is all great, but the reality is we need them so much more when it is all a mess.

PAUSE FOR THOUGHT

Let's take a moment to reflect on when you have felt a challenging emotion in the past: stress, overwhelm, anxiety, loneliness, comparison . . . whatever it may be, then ask yourself:

- How did you manage it? Maybe you managed it well, or perhaps it didn't go so well – just acknowledge this here too.
- How could you manage this feeling as a new mum if it crops up?

Your mind is a valuable, important resource and is central to your health and well-being. It will probably be tested on your journey through motherhood, so taking time to protect and nurture it is vital.

Your physical needs are also easy to forget as a new mum, but your postpartum body is changed and needs caring for as well, so we are going to delve into this in the next chapter.

REMEMBER:

- You must care for yourself to be the parent you wish to be to your baby. Feel no guilt in meeting your needs too.
- Communication within your support network is key in this time. Vocalise how you are feeling and how you need them to help you improve this.
- Know that if you are experiencing PND there is professional help available and accessing it is a sign of strength not weakness.

20

THE TRUTH ABOUT YOUR POSTPARTUM BODY

Your body goes on a journey like no other through pregnancy and birth – the most monumental adventure and wild challenge. The physical changes during pregnancy and the postpartum will look different for every woman, but what we all have in common is a need to understand our postnatal selves, to respect our bodies and to allow rehabilitation and recovery to happen with compassion and patience.

Before we delve any further, there is one way every single postpartum mum should be described and that is as an absolute superhero. Yet women are often left feeling like their postpartum body is something they need to cover up or be on a mission to change – that exact same body that has just made, nurtured, grown and birthed a whole new human life. We need to respect postpartum bodies; try to love your body for the journey it has been on and be super proud of yourself.

You are a strong, beautiful warrior.

I am relentlessly passionate about pelvic health and postnatal rehabilitation and, in this chapter, I want to share some of the immediate expectations and realities of your physical postpartum self, from top to toe.

> *Having always had a troubled relationship with my body, I thought I was going to struggle with pregnancy and birth. Through being informed, I had a positive birth experience and gained a whole new level of respect for my body. I have never been more proud to be a woman and never felt more in tune with the body which brought my baby into the world. I feel empowered.*
>
> Jessica

I will confess that, while I personally felt comfortable with the appearance of my postpartum body, I was shocked by the loss of strength despite being active and strength-training throughout my pregnancy. I thought at that point, *Wow, if I, as a midwife and pre- and postnatal trainer, am surprised by this huge physiological change, it is definitely taking a lot of us by surprise, so let's get talking about it more.*

I think there is a reason we often see one proud new parent walking out of the hospital, car seat in hand, but not the woman who has just birthed this precious new life. Zoom in and there she is, with supersized pads stuffed in her oversized knickers, supporting a stomach that feels all sorts of odd, shuffling down the corridor like her vagina might fall out at any minute. I remember it well! But it is exactly that postpartum reality that we have been notoriously bad at discussing honestly that has led to our postnatal selves being such a shock.

Your body will look and feel different in the postpartum. Being aware of some of the things that are common, what to expect and ways to support your body in this period can be really helpful so you are not taken by surprise at how you may look and feel, and you can feel confident about what is normal.

'I made a human, I am a superhero.'

POSTPARTUM POSTURE

When you are pregnant, your posture changes as your bump grows, and often this leads to flared ribs, a tilted pelvis and slumped shoulders. A tired new mum who is feeding and carrying a new baby can easily continue with this posture for months, and even years, to come, leading to weaknesses and injury. And, let's be honest, mums do not have time for being injured! I recommend taking note of your posture at little intervals throughout the day and making small efforts to bring your shoulders back, neutralise your pelvis and soften your knees. Use the posture diagram on page 59 as a handy reminder to perform a quick body scan. Taking some time to stretch your body, particularly your back and shoulders, can give instant relief and help prevent injury.

Another great, simple tool you can use to help rehabilitate your postpartum self is to practise breathing using your diaphragm:

- Lie down on a sofa or bed and place your hands around your rib cage.
- Take a deep inhale and allow your tummy and rib cage to expand into your hands.
- On your exhale, relax back to resting.

Breathing in this way has lots of benefits: it improves relaxation, improves strength and stability in your diaphragm and core muscles, and improves pelvic floor function.

YOUR BREASTS

Changes to your breasts postpartum may be more marked if you are breastfeeding your baby. As we discussed in Chapter 18, your breasts become large, hard and full (engorged) when your milk comes in and this typically coincides with the baby blues period discussed in Chapter 19, causing emotion and discomfort simultaneously which, although temporary, can be a tough time.

All women's breasts respond differently in pregnancy and breastfeeding, and while some may go relatively unchanged, others may increase in size dramatically. Bras are key to your comfort and breast health, and being measured is the best way to ensure a good size and fit. It is great to have done this in pregnancy; however, you are likely to find your size changes postnatally too, especially with breastfeeding, so being measured and ensuring you have a well-fitting and easy-access nursing bra will make your postnatal life feel much more comfortable. A bra that is too tight may be uncomfortable and can lead to blocked ducts, so a good fit with support but that is not restrictive is key.

YOUR TUMMY

When your baby is born, your uterus is still far larger than it was pre-pregnancy (five to six times in fact) and it doesn't immediately shrink back into your pelvis. It takes time. As a result, you may find you still look pregnant, but your uterus bump is much softer than your baby bump and mums often describe it as feeling jelly-like – soft but empty. The bounce-back stomach postpartum is a myth (no matter what you might see on social media) and our bodies need to be slowly nurtured back, not rushed.

The other difference postpartum that mums may notice is diastasis recti or a 'gap' down the middle of their tummy. A diastasis is a normal change that happens to all women in pregnancy. The rectus abdominis muscles run parallel to each other down the midline of your tummy and are joined together in the middle by connective tissue called the linea alba. During pregnancy, these two muscles move apart, and the linea alba tissue stretches to accommodate your growing baby. For many women, this naturally heals postpartum, but for others, they will need additional rehabilitation to help resolve it. It is estimated than over one-third of women at 12 months still have a diastasis recti.

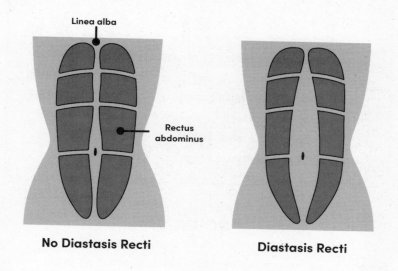

Linea alba

Rectus abdominus

No Diastasis Recti   **Diastasis Recti**

There are many things we can do to support this reconnection and healing process, from the diaphragmatic breathwork discussed earlier to gentle core awareness and reconnection exercises in the early postpartum. You can begin early core engagement exercises as early as you feel you would like to and feel comfortable to postpartum, and they are safe for all types of birth. Scan the QR code on page 6 for a video demo of these exercises.

TIGER STRIPES OR 'MUMMY MARKS'

Your skin has made huge changes to accommodate your little one and its elasticity is really tested along the way. Stretch marks are very common in pregnancy, affecting around 80 per cent of women, and they can vary in colour from red, pink, purple or brown depending on the colour of your skin. The most common places stretch marks are found are on your stomach, thighs and breasts, and they occur as a result of the dermis, the middle layer of skin, becoming broken as the skin stretches. Although excessive weight gain does increase the chance of stretch marks in pregnancy, the likelihood of getting them is otherwise thought to be down to genetics and your individual skin make-up. Often they fade once your baby is born, but they do not always disappear. There are many creams claiming to prevent stretch marks, but there is no conclusive evidence that they will make a significant difference.

WOUNDS

Some tearing or trauma to the vaginal, perineal or anal area is common after birth, affecting 85–90 per cent of women who give birth vaginally. The 25 per cent of women who give birth abdominally by caesarean section will have an abdominal wound. When your placenta comes away post-birth, it also leaves a wound about the size of a dinner plate on your uterus. This means that the vast majority of women's postpartum bodies have a wound that requires healing, and this is another reason why the postpartum body needs time and rehabilitation to repair.

If we were to undergo injury in another aspect of life or a form of surgery (a perineal repair is a surgical procedure, and a caesarean section is major abdominal surgery), you would expect to do exercises to rehabilitate and for the process to take time. You would also focus on rest, sleep and nutrition. Where postpartum recovery is so unique is that your body is in an acute phase of recovery, but you are also typically in chronic sleep deprivation, embarking on the huge challenge of learning how to care for a new baby, and are at risk of anaemia from bleeding and nutritional deficiencies from often not prioritising this in the fourth trimester.

We don't have a magic wand to suddenly improve postpartum sleep and there will always be days when you are trapped under a sleeping baby and you grab a lunch of biscuits (chocolate Hobnobs were my favourite). But, what we *can* do is have an awareness of what journey our body is going on and why we need to consider our own needs when we see them start to slide down the priority list. I am never going to tell a new mum to put the biscuits down, but what I do encourage is focusing on consuming adequate protein – an important macronutrient – as this is fundamental to wound and tissue healing. Normally you need around 0.75g/kg/day (52.5g protein/day for a 70-kg woman), but increasing protein to 1.8–1.9g/kg/day (126–133g protein/day for a 70-kg woman) has been shown to improved wound healing, and extra protein has been shown to be important in breastfeeding mums too. Below are some examples of protein-rich foods you can prepare ahead of time to snack on – I've included the grams of protein so you can see how to build it to get your daily requirement:

- 1 cooked chicken breast = 55g protein
- 1 egg = 6g protein
- 3 tablespoons lentils = 9g protein
- 3 tablespoons baked beans = 6g protein

- 100g tofu = 8g protein
- 30g peanuts = 8g protein
- 200ml milk = 8g protein
- 150ml yoghurt = 8g protein
- 30g cheese = 8g protein

Some women may also choose to supplement with protein snack bars or powders, which can give you a convenient 20g protein on average.

Keeping infection at bay is an important factor in promoting wound healing, and allowing your wound to get air, when possible, is crucial as typically postpartum wounds are in a sweaty area that increases the risk of bacteria growth. Good hand hygiene and wiping your vagina from front to back, not back to front as this can introduce bacteria in or around your anus into a perineal or vaginal wound, can also really help.

Having a regular (every couple of days) look at your perineal or caesarean wound in the early weeks is a good idea for monitoring your recovery and for observing for any signs of infection. If you notice increasing redness, pus-like discharge, an offensive smell, increased bleeding or a sudden increase in pain or should you feel unwell or feverish at any point, it is important to contact your midwife or GP as this may indicate an infection. You may feel a little anxious or squeamish about looking at your wound for the first time, so it is absolutely fine to have someone – whether that is your partner, midwife or health visitor – support you with this.

YOUR PELVIC FLOOR

In the postpartum period, your pelvic floor is usually in its most compromised state, and it may take a little time to reconnect with the same sensation you had when performing your pelvic floor exercises pre- or during pregnancy. But please do persevere – it is an essential part of your postpartum rehabilitation to reduce your risk of complications such as incontinence and prolapse.

Aim to start your pelvic floor exercises as soon as possible after birth. If you have had a catheter inserted into your bladder, wait for this to be removed before starting. For a refresh on how to perform these, head back to page 65. The reality is that 50 per cent of postpartum women live with a pelvic organ prolapse and 34 per cent with urinary incontinence. These statistics are too high and we really need to shake the taboo around pelvic health. Pregnant and postpartum women are more susceptible to pelvic floor dysfunction and educating yourself on pelvic health as well as developing that reconnection with your pelvic floor is an important protective factor to reducing your risk.

Clare Bourne, pelvic floor physiotherapist @clarebournephysio and author of *Strong Foundations*, has written some of her expert tips for you post-birth here:

During the early hours and days after birth, your body can feel very sore, painful and alien to you. It will improve, I promise, but know that you are not alone in how you are feeling and it can feel quite worrying. Here are some top tips to help you navigate those early days.

Top tips after vaginal delivery

1. *Sit on two rolled-up towels under your thighs to reduce any pressure on your perineum or any stitches you might have. This helps to reduce discomfort and pain when sitting down.*
2. *Use a cold pack on your perineum to reduce swelling and pain. The best way to do this is get a maternity pad and wet it with water, pop it in the freezer and, once frozen, wrap it completely in an old towel and pop it over your perineum for 5–10 minutes. You can repeat this every few hours.*

3. *Wash the perineum during each wee. If you have stitches or a graze from birth that is healing this can be really sore and painful when you do a wee. Therefore, take a cup of water with you and flush your vulva with water during or just after doing a wee. This can help to reduce any discomfort felt.*

Top tips after caesarean delivery

1. *Support your scar when you cough, sneeze or laugh. Place both hands over your wound and apply a gentle pressure. This can help to reduce discomfort.*
2. *To get out of bed, roll onto your side, let your feet drop off the side of the bed and, as they go down, push yourself up with your arms. This is the best way to get up. Do the reverse to get back in. This technique aims to reduce how much you have to use your tummy and therefore helps reduce pain.*
3. *Little bits of movement can help manage pain in the early days and reduce inflammation. Therefore, with the support and under the guidance of the medical team, getting out of bed on the day of your caesarean or early the next day is advised.*

I cannot recommend enough getting a postnatal Mummy MOT check. A Mummy MOT is a specialist postnatal examination for women following both vaginal and C-section births. It assesses how your posture, pelvic floor muscles and stomach muscles are recovering. Check out the Further Resources section on page 311 for the website to find your local practitioners.

PEES, POOS AND PILES

Often women on the labour ward tell me that they are really worried about the dreaded first pee or poo, and then they go and realise it wasn't so bad after all!

If you have had a vaginal birth, it is often concentrated urine that may cause a stinging sensation, so ensuring you're well-hydrated so your urine is more watery and less concentrated, and even peeing in the bath, shower or while pouring water over the area for the first time, can help.

Not delaying your first poop is also important. When you get the urge to go, it is important you do go at that time otherwise the poop retreats back up the digestive tract, leaving a harder, drier poop that may be more uncomfortable to pass. A fibre-rich diet and adequate hydration are key factors in ensuring your poop is soft and easy to pass, as well as being much kinder on your pelvic floor. You want to avoid pushing and/or straining to get a poo out as this may put extra pressure on your healing perineal or abdominal wound, and also puts additional strain on your pelvic floor when it is at its most vulnerable. Using the downwards breath (see page 48) is great as well as elevating your feet on a small step or stool so your knees are slightly higher than your hips and resting your forearms on your thighs (Emma Brockwell's tips for pelvic health in pregnancy on page 69 are also transferable and important postnatally).

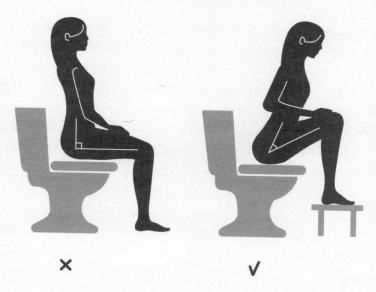

X   ✓

Piles or haemorrhoids are often a concern for postpartum women and are very common after birth. These are swollen blood vessels in and around the anus which can be itchy and sometimes painful too. Preventing constipation and practising your pelvic floor exercises will both help to prevent and resolve piles. If you have piles that do not resolve in the early postpartum, speak with your GP who can advise you on options for creams and treatments.

PAUSE FOR THOUGHT

What steps can you take in the early postpartum to help your body recover, re-nourish and repair? It could be easy, ready-to-go high-protein snack ideas, pelvic floor reminders or getting your poop step ready.

There is also a postnatal survival tool on page 306 which will bring all of this together.

By sharing some of these common realities, I am not telling you that your postpartum body is weak – far from it. I believe your postpartum self can be your strongest and most capable version . . . I mean, look at what you have achieved! But we must recognise that your postpartum body does need you to be compassionate and understanding, and this can only be achieved through information about your physiology because, whatever way you birth your baby, there are injuries to be rehabilitated.

REMEMBER:

- Early diaphragmatic breathing, pelvic floor exercises and gentle core engagement are safe and beneficial to your recovery.
- A caesarean birth is major abdominal surgery through seven different layers of tissue. It is therefore important to be patient and take your time to recover and nourish your body.
- 'Bounce-back' is a myth and your body deserves compassion and respect for its journey.

PART 3
REFLECTION

My hope in this part of the book is that it will help you enter parenthood with some of the key information you need to get off to a calmer, smoother start. There is a balance when talking about the immediate postpartum because there are often elements of overwhelming love and gratitude intertwined with huge change, new and difficult emotions, and significant physical healing. I remember feeling conflicted between times of wanting to soak up every moment and feeling a level of anxiety I had never known before, all speckled with incredible love and yet simultaneous feelings of loneliness. Whatever raw emotions you may find yourself navigating, please know you are not alone on this journey.

You are now equipped with key information about caring for yourself and your new baby in the hours and first days of parenthood, and there is a whole spectrum of what normal looks like during this time. Some babies sleep a lot, others do not and often your baby seeks your arms as a safe space to rest among the new and strange world they have been born into. Soak up the memories when you can and protect your newborn bubble, only letting in things or people who help and bring joy rather than adding to the demands of your life at this time. In the harder moments, use breathwork tools to ground and calm yourself, knowing this phase will pass and lighter times are ahead.

Quiz

Our third and final quiz is here. Give these questions a go to test your new post-birth knowledge.

1. What is the initial hour after birth called?
2. What is the vitamin offered to your baby post-birth?
3. How many wet nappies should your baby have in the first 24 hours minimum?
4. How many dirty nappies should your baby have in the first 24 hours minimum?
5. What macronutrient is key for healing postpartum?
6. How common is urinary incontinence postpartum?
7. How common is the baby blues?
8. How common is postnatal depression?

The quiz answers are on page 309 so you can check your new knowledge.

Jot down any key take-homes from Part 3 in the space below:

_____

_____

_____

_____

_____

_____

_____

A FINAL MESSAGE

As we reach the end of this book, I want you to know that it has been a privilege to hold your hand through these pages as you prepare for your baby's arrival into the world. As you continue through your final days, weeks or months of pregnancy and transition into the world of motherhood, these pages are still here for you. Come back to them whenever you need to feel empowered and understood.

I want to remind you that you are more capable than you realise and stronger than you know. I encourage you along this journey to allow yourself to recognise and acknowledge your strength and abilities, vocalise them and celebrate them. Women are phenomenal and I am blessed to witness just how amazing women's bodies and babies are in my practice as a midwife – you are incredible.

I know there may be hurdles or twists and turns in the road as you approach labour and birth, but know that you do not need to fear these bumps. You have all the tools within you to navigate them and remain on a path to a positive and empowered birth. We must always remember that there is no best way to birth; there are endless variations of labour and birth and yours will be unique to you. Birth is not an event to compare, it is your own journey, and all births can leave you feeling positive and empowered.

The incredibly wise words of midwife Ina May Gaskin sum up the importance of your birth experience: '*Whenever and however you give birth, your experience will impact your emotions, your mind, your body, and your spirit for the rest of your life.*'

We have been on an intimate journey through this book. You have considered much yourself and trusted in my expertise and experience as a midwife to guide you. I have been where you are now, preparing to give birth or having recently just done so, pondering over what it may look like and wondering how I will bring my baby into the world or adapt to the new role of being a mum. As a result, I have experienced first-hand the value of being empowered and informed, and my knowledge led me to have a birth experience I will forever look back on with ear-to-ear smiles. I will always be in awe of what my body achieved through its 40 weeks and 2 days of pregnancy and in bringing our son safely into the world. The feelings I had following my birth were a real motivator behind creating this book for you, because every woman should feel proud and powerful when they birth, however they may birth.

A key part of my own birth preparation, and something I encourage all expectant mothers to do, was to read positive birth stories as I prepared for birth. I never intended on sharing my own birth story. It is such a personal, precious journey, but fitting with my ethos of supporting women to be excited for birth, not scared, I feel it is important I share it with you. It is raw and real and my final tool to support you in your positive birth journey.

MY BIRTH STORY: WATER BIRTH

17 September 2021: the most amazing and empowering day of my life. The day our son was born.

The day before Finley's birth, I went to see our community midwife for a stretch and sweep. We had tried two days before, but my cervix was too posterior, and Finley's head was too low for it to be successful. So, first note here is to not be disheartened if you too have an unsuccessful stretch and sweep, partly because the evidence for their success isn't there and partly because, just a couple of days later, it was successful, my cervix was 3cm dilated and my waters broke. I would call that progress! For which I was mega grateful as, like many women who watch their due date come and go, I was feeling a little (very) impatient.

I can't say I was contracting at this point; some niggly period-style pains were all. But I knew how I could support my body for this next stage: a nourishing dinner, walks with my husband, ball bouncing, hydration, creating a calm oxytocin-promoting environment and then some sleep.

Not a full night, mind . . . roll on 2am and contractions began.

I tiptoed out of bed telling my husband I couldn't sleep and was going to watch a film in the living room. In my experience, a tired birth partner isn't optimal, and it wasn't a total fib because I did put a film on – I can't even remember what it was, but some easy-going romcom. I bounced, paced, lunged, swayed my hips, breathed (A LOT of this!), lit my favourite candles, had some toast and sipped water until my husband must have become suspicious and joined me at around 5.30am. By which time I couldn't disguise these powerful waves of contractions that were coming every few minutes. There was lots more moving around by me. From helping optimise your baby's position, opening your pelvis and being a great form of pain relief, mobility is your friend for sure! Hydration and nutrition were in full swing thanks to my husband and on went my TENS machine.

A couple more hours went by and my husband was becoming increasingly worried about hitting traffic on the way to the hospital. The car journey was somewhat uncomfortable so distraction was key! We sang Rag'n'Bone Man songs at the tops of our voices all the way there and I can't promise it sounded pretty, but it helped and must have helped boost my endorphins. I don't know about you, but I was up for maximising these bad boys as much as possible, even if I sounded more like a strangled cat than Rag'n'Bone Man.

A few stops along the corridor, more hip swaying and deep breathing, and we arrived at the birthing centre and were greeted by our midwife, an incredible friend of mine who came in to care for us. My husband set about creating the birth environment we had discussed: music, lighting, diffuser, snack station, etc. Our focus was to make a space that was calming and relaxing to promote all the oxytocin and suppress adrenaline. My contractions were powerful and frequent, and I continued to embrace upright, forwards and open positions that felt natural and instinctive. Leaning forwards on a birthing ball on the floor was a favourite of mine at this stage.

Our midwife did all the important checks to make sure we were all well and safe to stay in the low-risk birthing setting. Good job we were because my husband had created the environment I had dreamed of pretty much since the day I saw those two lines on a pregnancy test. I am sure I'm not the only woman whose mind jumped nine months forwards after peeing on a stick (before the obvious shorter-term concerns then crept in, of course).

After a short time I opted to use the birthing pool. Ohhhhh my dipping into that was heavenly, the relief was wonderful. I had done a lot of swimming in pregnancy, and it reminded me of sinking into the pool on hols on swollen summer evenings and feeling instant relaxation.

In total, my labour was six hours long. At the time I thought I felt every one of those hours, but, looking back, I feel it zoomed by! I didn't stay in the pool for long on my initial dip, mainly because I vomited in it (not my proudest moment but a common side effect to labour!) and partly because after a further vaginal examination I opted to have a dose of pethidine. This allowed me to gain a bit of rest. Our little one was super low in my pelvis and, as a result, I was getting pelvic pain in between the contractions that didn't ease up. Having a couple of hours' respite was exactly what we needed. That being said, every time a contraction came I dashed from the snug side-lying position on a comfy beanbag to sit on the toilet! Toilets are popular places for women in labour and it was again an instinctive feeling to need to move and be there when each contraction came. The other great benefit was I stayed mobile throughout.

It turns out it was the hindwaters that broke the day before and my fore-waters were still intact providing a cushion between his head and my cervix. So our midwife broke these and I jumped (I was so desperate to get back in I don't think jump is far off!) back into the pool.

Finley, our beautiful boy, was born calmly in the water very soon after this. I was beyond blessed to lift him up onto my chest surrounded by the most kind, compassionate and supportive team. I cannot even begin to describe how I felt in that moment.

As a midwife fully aware of ALL the potential labour complications, I definitely felt a massive sense of relief.

As a mum, I felt completely overwhelmed with love for this tiny baby. An immense amount of love I never even knew was possible.

As a woman, I felt strong and proud of what my body had achieved, like I could take on the world. It was genuinely the most incredible and empowering day of my life.

I often talk about the potential twists and turns of labour and believe that, regardless of what a birth looks like for each individual, it should ALWAYS leave women feeling the way I was fortunate enough to on this day. This has only made me even more passionate to continue teaching my online courses.

There were a few twists in my own birth. I couldn't pass urine in labour – this is common, but it is really important that bladders are emptied. A full bladder can inhibit a baby descending in the birth canal, damage the muscles if overstretched and it is also important that urine output is measured to screen for dehydration in labour. I had a couple of catheters inserted to ensure my bladder was cared for. My placenta was also a bit stubborn to come out, so an obstetric consultant came to help it on its way. I thought I would love using Entonox (gas and air) – turns out it wasn't for me at all and made me nauseous despite having seen it work fantastically for many women in my care over the years. But none of this mattered; I was supported with compassion by the team with me, and made to feel safe and empowered to make informed choices throughout.

We cuddled up as a family, tucking into chilli con carne and sticky toffee pudding while Finley found his love of my milk in a bubble of amazement. A few hours later, we left the hospital in which I have spent many years working, but this time with our baby – ready to enter a new chapter of our lives encapsulated in a love like no other.

I could not be prouder to be a woman, a mum and a midwife.

YOUR POSTPARTUM
SURVIVAL TOOL

Everyone's well-being will be enhanced by different things – this is your space to plan what will help you in the postpartum.

There will inevitably be days or nights that feel tougher than others and that is because postpartum is hard, but you can do hard things and you're capable of more than you realise. Practising self-compassion and kindness doesn't come naturally to us all, but it really will be of benefit to your postpartum self, so I encourage you to fill in this little tool now so that you can reflect back on it when you need to.

On the challenging days I am going to remind myself that . . .

_____

_____

_____

_____

When I could do with some help I am going to ask . . .

_____

_____

_____

_____

_____

To protect my psychological well-being I will . . .

_____

_____

_____

To protect my physical well-being I will . . .

_____

_____

_____

These are the jobs I am going to delegate/skip when I don't have the time or energy for them . . .

_____

_____

_____

I will practise self-care and compassion by . . .

_____

_____

_____

_____

YOUR POSTNATAL
MOOD DIARY

This is your space for the first six weeks post-birth to grant yourself the compassion and respect to observe how you are feeling. Detecting low mood early, creating spaces and ways to support your mental well-being, and accessing help early if needed is so important. A mood diary is really helpful in this immediate postpartum space because it can help you keep an eye on any changes to your mood, and you may even notice that you have more positive mood days than you realise. This diary can also help you spot anything like activities, sleep quality or certain people that make you feel better or worse. Photocopy the tracker below so you can use it for those first six weeks post-birth.

Day of week	Mood (0–10)	Other mood details	Hours of sleep	Thought that triggered mood	Situation that triggered mood	What helped?
Sun						
Mon						
Tue						
Wed						
Thur						
Fri						
Sat						

QUIZ ANSWERS

Part 1

1. Upwards breath
2. Downwards breath
3. Approximately 60 seconds
4. Oxytocin
5. 32 weeks
6. 150 minutes
7. 36 weeks
8. The Scales and BRAIN tools

Part 2

1. Latent phase, first stage, transition, second stage, third stage
2. Adrenaline
3. UFOM

4. Consultant-led unit (also called labour ward or delivery suite)
5. Ventouse and forceps
6. 25 per cent
7. 34 weeks
8. 36 weeks

Part 3

1. The Golden Hour
2. Vitamin K
3. At least 1
4. At least 1
5. Protein
6. 34 per cent
7. 80 per cent
8. 10 per cent

FURTHER RESOURCES

Pregnancy and birth

See midwifepip.com for my full range of exclusive, expert-led online and live courses, on topics including pregnancy support, birth preparation, pregnancy exercise and preparing to breastfeed.

Websites
Birthrights: birthrights.org.uk
Group B Strep Support: gbss.org.uk
NHS Squeezy App: squeezyapp.com
The Twins Trust: twinstrust.org

Books
Strong Foundations by Clare Bourne (Thorsons, 2023)
The Science of Nutrition by Rhiannon Lambert (DK, 2021)

Products
The Wave Comb: www.thewavecomb.co.uk

Postpartum and parenthood

See midwifepip.com for my full range of postpartum care, including parenting, postnatal recovery and exercise courses, all led by experts and offering exceptional support every step of the way.

Websites
Birth Trauma Association: birthtraumaassociation.org.uk
The Breastfeeding Network: breastfeedingnetwork.org.uk
The Lullaby Trust: lullabytrust.org.uk
Mind: mind.org.uk
Mini First Aid: minifirstaid.co.uk
The Mummy MOT: themummyMOT.com
PANDAS Foundation UK: pandasfoundation.org.uk
UNICEF breastfeeding resources: unicef.org.uk/babyfriendly/
baby-friendly-resources/breastfeeding-resources/

Books
Why Did No One Tell Me? by Emma Brockwell (Vermilion, 2021)
The Just Chill Baby Sleep Book by Rosey Davidson (Vermilion, 2023)
The Little Book of Calm for New Mums by Anna Mathur (Penguin, 2022)
Mind Over Mother by Anna Mathur (Piatkus, 2020)

Products
Cheeky Wipes: cheekywipes.com
The Nappy Lady: thenappylady.co.uk

ACKNOWLEDGEMENTS

I want to take a moment here to acknowledge some of the incredible people who have supported and influenced the writing of this book, because without them it would not be in your hands today and influencing your birth.

First of all, thank you to the families and women who I have been honoured to support in my career as a midwife, to those following me on Instagram, listening to my podcast and joining me on my pregnancy and postnatal courses. Your influence, questions and honesty over your experiences were the motivation behind writing this book. You have driven my relentless passion to ensure that women have empowered, positive birthing experiences, regardless of any twists or turns; that appropriate medical intervention can be welcomed through informed decision-making and in the absence of fear; that birth can be a momentous event women feel calm, safe and confident to journey through; and that taboo topics are spoken about.

To the phenomenal team at Penguin Random House. To Sam Jackson who saw the capability in me to write this book and approached me to create it. Your belief in me provided me with the confidence to drive this forward. Evangeline Stanford, for supporting with making sure my medical brain could make sense to every reader and sorting my poor grammar. Julia Kellaway, who has tirelessly worked with me to make this book as good as it possibly can be and to ensure it can meet my intentions of helping every reader achieve a better, more positive birth. Thank you to the editing team for embracing my liberal word count so we could ensure this book covers all the detail women need to know in the depth they deserve. To the whole team behind the scenes and the illustrators for making my vison a reality and allowing this book to be so much more than merely a book to read, but a guide to empower.

To my book agent, Lauren Gardiner, who has not only shared my passion for this book, but has always been on hand to keep me on track and respond to my panicked voice notes with a calm, reassuring hand. You have been pivotal in making this journey possible.

To my husband, James, for mirroring my passion for improving families' experiences, cheerleading me through the tough times, picking me up when anxiety takes over and being my best friend through it all. I am not sure there is anyone else on this planet who could understand me and my goals, and stand beside me to achieve whatever I put my mind to in the way you do, day in and day out, and for that I will always be grateful. Known unofficially as 'tech-guy', your willingness to learn new skills so that I can palm all the tasks out of my direct expertise on to you is admirable and one of the reasons we are such a great team.

To my son Finley, who is too young to know how much he inspires me every day, brings me joy and sunshine when the days feel dark and keeps me present when my mind is muddled with the to-do list. To my second baby boy, Alfie, currently growing inside me as I write this book and reminding me how capable women are, motivating me as we expand our family to ensure others can do so in a supported and informed way too. Being your mummy will always be my greatest achievement and I am so blessed you chose me. I hope, above all, that my work and this book teach you to stay passionate, be bold and to go out there and achieve your dreams.

To my friends and family, who have tolerated my inability to respond to messages in the same week they were received – those who I have cancelled or rearranged plans on due to work commitments and deadlines, but who have understood, been at the end of the phone and supported me despite the lack of coffee dates. So many of you have shown immense kindness and true friendship which has made a huge difference to me on this book-writing journey, and I hope to repay you the same support.

To my mum and dad, who have helped shape me, allowed me to run wild with my stubborn ways and 'can-do' attitude to life and encouraged me to be ambitious.

To our midwife, Kate, who, in 2021, supported our son safely into the world and made me feel safe, respected, heard and powerful. Our family created memories that day that we will treasure forever, and the positive experience I felt personally has further motivated me to ensure women have the level of information and support they deserve as they prepare to birth their baby.

To the experts and women who have contributed to this book and shared their knowledge or personal experiences to help others, your support is invaluable, and I have endless thank yous to you all for contributing.

ABOUT THE AUTHOR

Pip began her midwifery journey in 2012 and has worked across a variety of settings gaining invaluable experience in various hospitals before becoming a midwifery sister on a diverse delivery suite in 2019. Pip continues to work as a practising midwifery sister in the NHS on a delivery suite supporting women through their birth journeys today.

Pip is passionate about continued education, being up to date and an expert in her field, which led her to being involved in published research and quality improvement projects, and to complete her master's degree with distinction in 2021 as well as training as a hypnobirthing teacher and pre- and postnatal exercise specialist.

Pip also has an interest in pelvic health and is completing work as a specialist pelvic health midwife through her additional training in this field while working privately to provide women with pelvic health and Mummy MOT postnatal checks that they deserve.

In 2021, Pip became increasingly frustrated seeing families poorly equipped with conflicting, inaccurate or unrealistic advice and information, and recognised that women deserved better. Pip believes passionately that, with the right support and honest and evidence-based information, all births should be positive regardless of any twists and turns that may crop up. For this reason, Pip began her Instagram page @midwife_pip followed by her podcast, *Midwife Pip Podcast*, and online courses (www.midwifepip.com), covering everything from pregnancy support in all three trimesters, to expert birth preparation, postpartum courses with the very best expert information and support, and specialist pre- and postnatal exercise programmes. Pip is on hand to support and guide women through all aspects of pregnancy, birth, postpartum and parenting milestones every step of the way so that all expectant and new mums feel like superwomen during pregnancy and when they give birth.

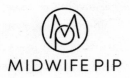

MIDWIFE PIP

INDEX